THE
PILLARS
OF HEALTH

ALSO BY JOHN PIERRE

Cooking DVDs

When Bachelor Meets Homemaker

Vegan Weight Loss

In the Kitchen with John Pierre and Friends

The Unprocessed 30 Day Challenge

Please visit:

Hay House USA: www.hayhouse.com®
Hay House Australia: www.hayhouse.com.au
Hay House UK: www.hayhouse.co.uk
Hay House South Africa: www.hayhouse.co.za
Hay House India: www.hayhouse.co.in

THE PILLARS OF HEALTH

Your Foundations for
Lifelong Wellness

JOHN PIERRE

HAY HOUSE, INC.
Carlsbad, California • New York City
London • Sydney • Johannesburg
Vancouver • Hong Kong • New Delhi

Library of Congress Cataloging-in-Publication Data (to come)

Hardcover ISBN: 978-1-4019-4220-5
Tradepaper ISBN: 978-1-4019-4222-9

16 15 14 13   4 3 2 1
1st edition, September 2013

Printed in the United States of America

*This book is dedicated to everyone
striving to make the world
a better place.*

CONTENTS

INTRODUCTION

My nutrition and fitness research began more than 30 years ago and gradually progressed to become my life's work. Fueled by my burning desire to help improve people's well-being, I studied countless health-enhancing modalities through seminars, classes, workshops, books, manuals, and scientific journals, and trained under doctors and other health practitioners. My goal was not to acquire a collection of diplomas, certifications, or licenses, nor did I seek to break the record of accumulated course-work hours. My philosophy simply centered on the belief that the more I learned, the more tools I would have to help people attain increased well-being.

As I began to share my knowledge and witness the profound benefits people experienced as a result, I was able to expand my understanding of the fundamental principles of health and assist even more individuals.

You could say that the spark that ignited this book occurred more than 25 years ago when both clients and attendees at my lectures began requesting written materials highlighting and summarizing the information I taught. They encouraged me to write a book so that they could take the ideas home with them as a source of additional motivation and guidance. As much as I wanted to provide supportive material to everyone immediately, my full schedule of traveling, lecturing, teaching, and volunteering simply didn't permit me the time to sit down and write. Instead, I took a few free minutes here and there to jot down critical information—notes that I wanted to compile into a helpful guide one day.

As the decades passed, I observed the continuing degradation of our planet, along with escalating health struggles for a large percentage of the population. It became increasingly important for me to get the information I had to a greater number of people. My heartfelt desire to reach and assist as many individuals as possible compelled me to finally complete the book you now hold.

It has been my overriding goal to make the information contained in these pages simple and straightforward to understand and apply, instead of getting caught up in tedious and confusing scientific and technical jargon. The principles of vibrant health are basic and easy (as they should be), and living them is pleasurable and sustaining (a big clue that you're on the path to success). This book will help guide you on an amazing journey with simple yet revolutionary approaches to wellness.

For years, I've been hearing new clients say, "I feel like I'm falling apart." It became clear that their lifestyle structures weren't solid. Instead of feeling sturdy and energetic, they often felt as though they were standing on frail pillars of sand. While they may have been doing well in certain areas, such as exercising, other areas were weakening because of detrimental dietary choices or negative mental habits.

To experience exceptional vitality and lasting energy well into our later years, it's important to learn how to strengthen the "pillars" which support our lives. These include a healthful diet, positive mental habits, physical movement that engages the body in challenging and fun ways, and a compassionate connection with ourselves and others. Just as pillars are used to reinforce architectural structures, when we strengthen our health foundations, we thrive in fantastic ways.

The book is divided into four parts, each of which focuses on topics that relate to establishing a vibrant, solid health base. If pillars are needed to hold up a building, what happens when one or two are damaged or removed? The structure will weaken and may collapse. Similarly, when you reinforce your health pillars, you stand a better chance of holding up the sound structure of your body, mind, and spirit, while contributing positively to loved ones and the community around you.

Part I, The Pillar of Nutrition, explains the physiological and emotional reasons processed foods are detrimental. The trend over the past millennium has moved toward consuming denatured ingredients that cannot sustain optimal human functioning. Understanding the fundamentals of eating that promote vibrant energy will inspire you to look at food in new ways and make more informed decisions in choosing meals. It's those "Aha!" moments that will shake you out of poor dietary habits. This section delivers thought-provoking revelations that will help you make more positive, whole-food choices.

In Part II, The Pillar of Mind, you'll learn why creativity, nutritional support, and sufficient rest are all essential building blocks for a fully functioning brain. The ideas, techniques, and suggestions in these chapters will help sustain and improve your cognitive abilities for optimal performance.

Currently, many who engage in standard exercise routines are bored, unmotivated, and injury-prone. Part III, The Pillar of Motion, will help you break free from the negative effects of prolonged sitting and release you from the "hibernation" cycle. There's tremendous creativity and joy in movement; you just need to remember to invite your most neglected ally—fun. The numerous suggestions and photos in these chapters will motivate everyone to move more.

The last section, Part IV: The Pillar of Compassion, will encourage you to listen to your caring internal voice. A solid foundation of trusting yourself with confidence will help support your empathy, honor, and kindness. You'll learn the importance of using kind words with yourself and others and how to cultivate the attitude of compassion and focus on the positive.

This book conveys in very simple, understandable, and doable ways that whole foods, a creative mind, a strong body, and a compassionate conscience create a win-win scenario for everyone. By following the principles I describe, you'll build a solid foundation for yourself, humanity, and the planet by encouraging, sustaining, and supporting your true nature—love.

PART I

THE PILLAR OF NUTRITION

CHAPTER 1

SHAKY NUTRITIONAL FOUNDATIONS

Since humans first inhabited the earth, survival has been our genetic drive. Next to air, water, and shelter, adequate nourishment was crucial for the continued existence of our species. From nature's point of view, storing reserve energy as body fat was a necessary safeguard that ensured we'd have the potential to live another day and hopefully procreate. Nature never worried that we'd get so "lucky" as to become obese.

Long ago, loss of life frequently came from starvation, injuries, infections, or predators. In modern times, the greatest causes of death are from diseases that have direct dietary correlations, namely the overconsumption of processed foods and animal products. Nutritious whole foods are readily available, but we're frequently choosing to fill up on processed foods that don't nourish us and add to our toxic load instead.

The most unhealthful diet is the one we're currently consuming—or is it now consuming us? Even though members of previous generations experienced food scarcity, their meals were spared from rivers of pesticides, cups of food additives, and syringes of hormones and bottles of antibiotics (which are routinely administered to farm animals). They enjoyed food in its whole, unprocessed form. In the not-so-distant past, only indulgent monarchs suffered from ailments such as obesity, diabetes, heart disease, and gout; but since many people can eat like royalty nowadays, they, along with small children, find themselves in the same disastrous health predicament.

Food provides fuel for more than just the body—it's a powerful social anchor that allows us to celebrate events with family and friends. Eating should be enjoyable and satisfying, but it must also supply nutritional value and contribute the vital components we need for excellent bodily function.

Today, you face several challenges that make nourishing yourself properly more difficult. In this chapter, I'll address the major roadblocks that obstruct you from eating healthfully and you'll gain a better understanding of why the modern diet is undermining cellular health.

Health Begins at the Cellular Level

Similar to pillars made of brick that serve as support for a building, human cells are the building blocks of the body. They make up our tissues, organs, glands, and bones—they form our entire structure and undergo constant construction and repair. Just as not having enough bricks or using inferior materials leads to weak infrastructure in a building, denying our cells critical macro- and micronutrients also affects their state of well-being. In addition, if we injure our cells with harmful chemicals and toxic substances, they will become unstable and damaged. This is often called disease.

Think of the body's cells as complex mini-factories where millions of microscopic, life-sustaining processes take place continually. If everything runs effectively, health and vitality is the result. That's why it's essential to provide the cells with the necessary biological building blocks that ensure optimal functioning. If we want the body to be sturdy and strong, we need to supply it generously with essential nutrients that create and maintain a solid foundation, while simultaneously reducing internal and external damage.

Vitamins, minerals, protein, carbohydrates, fat, oxygen, and phytonutrients or phytochemicals (bioactive plant-derived compounds associated with positive health effects, including anti-aging) ensure that cells perform their tasks at ideal levels. Just as important, some of these nutrients help protect the body's trillions of cells from the harmful attacks of the dangerous free radicals that bombard us constantly. These rogue molecules can cause premature aging and cellular destruction if not kept in check.

Ensuring that cells are properly hydrated and "bathed" in nutrients supplies them with the protective cellular surveillance and powerful safeguards they need to keep free radicals contained and immobilized. That's why the foods we choose to eat are so important. What we ingest can directly assist or harm our cells—food has the power to be either an antagonistic adversary or our helpful ally.

In the coming sections, I'll discuss the dangers of processed foods and you'll learn why many of the choices available today are simply masquerading as "impostor foods." Empowered with this newfound knowledge, you'll be able to make more informed choices about what you choose to invite into your diet for optimal health and well-being.

Living in Processville

In our abundant modern society, we've begun to use food for more than just survival. Through technology and science, agribusiness has revolutionized our way of eating, integrating processed foods deep into what we perceive as normal and accepted.

Many of today's children think that food comes from a box or bottle because they've been indoctrinated practically since birth into eating processed foods. It's become common to see infants fed formula right out of cans and plastic packages. As a result, children's taste buds become numbed from an early age with highly degraded, chemically modified, and unnaturally seasoned edibles.

Since most kids don't know what food in its natural state tastes like, when they try some wholesome fare, they're often disappointed by the subtle flavors. Their taste buds keep looking for the familiar chemical enhancers found in salty chips, sweet cookies, and gooey pizza because they've developed a "hyper palate," and so have many adults. Consequently, they avoid the comparatively mild flavors of whole foods.

It's like driving a car on the expressway at 65 miles per hour, then suddenly exiting onto a side street and slowing down to 20 miles per hour—it feels as if we're barely moving anymore. Similarly, our taste sensitivity decreases as we become used to processed foods, until the more subtle flavors of whole foods barely register.

Confusion abounds about what's good for us to eat, and it's no surprise. Our educational system fails to teach us about the greatest common denominator affecting our health: real food. Instead, we're encouraged to take eating for granted and use it as entertainment or emotional medication for sadness, boredom, and depression. This minimizes food's powerful value and stops us from seeing the bigger picture between what's on our plate and the fate of our health. Further exacerbating the situation, processed-food manufacturers take advantage of our ignorance by pushing their products on us with brain-surgeon precision.

There's a reason that unsuspecting youngsters demand those rainbow-colored boxes (which often contain a prize) with pictures of the latest cartoon or movie characters. Advertisers have analyzed both children's and adults' triggers and know exactly how to push them. Commercials have become virtual masterpieces of food seduction that hypnotize children into endlessly nagging their parents for another box of "sugar blitz" cereal or "macaroni and yellow goo."

Expertly designed processed-food packages are all around, mesmerizing us. Processed foods in bags and boxes have seductive qualities since they don't allow us to see what we're eating or, often, how much.

The repercussions of living in Processville are all too easy to see. Addiction to convenience and processed food has led our nation to disastrous results: Close to 70 percent of Americans are overweight, and sadly, the numbers are projected to increase dramatically over time.[1] Turning away from natural whole foods comes with a high price. Are we willing to continue paying it with our health?

Superseding Nature

It's hard to imagine that something as seemingly innocent as food can be turned into an addictive substance, but it can—and you're about to learn how.

Processed food manufacturers and their expertly trained staff understand our body chemistry well. Some employ more biochemists than dietitians. They know that portions of our brain respond to the combination of fat, sugar, and salt by experiencing an extreme "high." This is the reason they modify their laboratory creations with every imaginable taste enhancer, many of which are downright dangerous and even carcinogenic.[2] They often use the cheapest preservatives available, along with any chemicals they can get away with, to keep us coming back for more.

Our natural preferences for sweet, salty, and fatty foods are being routinely exploited. Manufacturers refine once-natural foods that grow from the earth and remove their water, fiber, and nutrients. Then the new concoction is revamped with dangerous oils, salt, sweeteners, artificial flavors, and artificial colors. We end up with potions nature never intended us to ingest.

Transforming whole foods into unnaturally rich, high-calorie "foods" starves us of micronutrients, fattens us up, and makes us more vulnerable to dietary-related diseases and cognitive decline. Processed foods dramatically alter our brain chemistry,[3] hormone levels, vitality, and ultimately, our very destiny.

Our taste buds and every cell in the body react to processed foods in addictive and detrimental ways.[4] Manufacturers enhance these drug-like effects by manipulating their formulas to keep us coming back for more. They guard their secret recipes like nuclear launch codes because billions of dollars in profits are at stake.

Food advertisers entice us all to buy "happiness" as short-term taste pleasure but conveniently fail to remind us of the long-term pain associated with dietary-related diseases such as diabetes, obesity, attention deficit disorder (ADD), hyperactivity, heart disease, and depression.

When scientists visit regions of the world where people still live in more primitive conditions and introduce processed foods like candy bars, soda, and fast foods, these individuals who were once living happy, addiction-free lives, soon become junk-food devotees. Because chemically tweaked foods supersede nature by hijacking the primal pleasure centers in the brain, we're no longer satisfied by just an apple or a handful of almonds. We become used to the stimulation of being pushed into the stratosphere, going far beyond what nature ever intended, entering a state of hyper-excitement that keeps us coming back for more.

Who runs out of the house at midnight for broccoli or carrots? But we gladly get into the car at crazy hours and drive to pick up pizza, soda, candy bars, chips, and ice cream because the alchemists of "hocus-pocus" foods have worked their sorcery.

Insatiable Hunger, Unquenchable Thirst

Since hunger dominated much of human history and food scarcity was the rule rather than the exception, nature programmed our brain to seek out energy-dense foods and rewarded us with "bonuses" for consuming them.

Some of these bonuses come as releases of brain opioids that encourage pleasant feelings of relief, relaxation, or enjoyable stimulation.[5] In the past, these biological responses ensured our survival. Today, manufacturers have turned them into health liabilities by consistently ringing the "pleasure doorbells" of our mind with chemically modified "foods."

Opioids carve out pathways in our brain when we eat or even *think* of highly palatable foods.[6] This is nature's way of helping us to seek and recognize concentrated edibles in the far-off future. But what happens when that distant future occurs every few hours as we eat breakfast, lunch, dinner, and snacks? We're rewarded with highs all day long instead of on rare occasions. This unnatural situation turns us into processed-food junkies. Instead of satisfying true nutritional demands, processed foods infused with salt, fat, artificial colors and flavors, and sugar alter our brain chemistry in ways that compel us to overeat[7] by encouraging our brain to crave more of the same high-calorie fare.

Our stomach has stretch receptors, and we also have nutrient receptors that monitor how much we've eaten to signal the brain when we feel full. Since refined foods condense hundreds of calories into small, unsatisfying portions, even if we consume more than enough, the brain doesn't get the signal to stop eating. It's tricked into thinking we're still hungry, and *overeating* becomes the only way to feel satisfied. The brain becomes neurally confused from continually consuming strange, high-calorie fatty mixtures not found in nature. After eating, the empty plate sitting before us tells us that we should have had enough, but our brain keeps thinking about what's left in the refrigerator or cupboards.

Most processed foods contain oil for a very important reason: It's a cheap flavor and texture enhancer. Our body uses components of most vegetable oils to make its own version of psychoactive ingredients.[8] Since a high percentage of desserts, sweets, and most processed foods contain added oils, our appetite is heightened. Eating two tablespoons of oil at 238 calories and 28 grams of fat won't appease our hunger for a minute. (I'll discuss oil in greater detail later in the book.) However, eating the same amount of calories in green leafy vegetables (that's almost two pounds) will not only satiate us quite nicely for some time but will also provide us with abundant antioxidants and phytochemicals.

The secret to feeling full after eating is ensuring adequate fiber, water, and nutrient intake. The water and fiber in whole foods provide crucial bulk and are one of the reasons my clients have lost up to 150 pounds in approximately one year (as noted by their physicians). I'll share which whole foods provide the best nutrient content in the next chapter.

The majority of clients I see today are greatly lacking in water. When our bodies are healthy, they're about 70 percent water. When we eat dry, processed foods such as bagels, cookies, and other packaged goods, they absorb the water in our body, much the way eating a sponge would.

When we're dehydrated, the blood thickens. Its consistency starts to resemble slow-moving maple syrup rather than quick-flowing grape juice, and our blood cells stop operating adequately. Immune cells cease doing their job effectively because they must inefficiently swim through sludge. Red blood cells, which carry oxygen, are impeded, leading to fatigue and lethargy.

Dehydration often sends our body in search of colorful, fizzy drinks filled with more chemicals instead of plain, clean water. Since we're used to the overpowering taste sensations of processed foods, our hyper palate motivates us to reach for bubbly concoctions, which continue to artificially stimulate our taste buds and brain while failing to quench our body's need for healthy liquids.

It's easy to mistake thirst signals for hunger as well, and we often reach out for more refined foods as a result. Because processed foods contain significantly fewer nutrients and have less volume, particularly less water and fiber, we're forced to consume more calories and toxins. Our nutritional demands are rarely satiated, and dehydration is frequently the norm rather than the exception. But wait—there's more.

Digestive Gridlock

When whole foods are refined, the process strips them of fiber, robbing us of this crucial material vital to our well-being. Those who suffer from foul breath frequently have elimination problems because of a lack of fiber in the diet. I've worked with many clients who experienced only one bowel movement during the week and who also suffered from severe acne and horrific lethargy. Processed foods and animal products were largely to blame.

Fiber affects bowel health and hormone function, assisting with removing harmful toxins, much like cleaning up a chemical spill.[9] It soaks up the undesirable substances and carries them out with the waste. If we're not supplying adequate fiber through our diet, it becomes difficult for the body to escort toxins out, and they can get absorbed back into the bloodstream.

The longer chemical poisons (particularly the antibiotics, hormones, pesticides, and concentrated heavy metals found in many animal products) sit in the intestinal tract, the greater the potential for harm. If the main channels of elimination are clogged up with toxic waste due to slow transit times, we risk damaging and altering cellular health. This is what makes constipation particularly dangerous.

Imagine what would happen if we put the trash outside weekly for pickup and the company responsible for its removal simply brought it back into the house and dumped it in the kitchen. What if this continued to happen every week for months? How would our house look and smell? The typical SAD (Standard American Diet) is dominated by fiberless animal products and processed foods, the magnets of constipation. The U.S. Department of Health and Human Services estimates that $725 million are spent on laxative products each year in the U.S. alone,[10] a predictable result of poor dietary choices.

All plants grown in nature contain ample fiber, while animal products don't have a speck. When I added whole plant foods to my clients' diet and they began to exercise, their bowels started functioning normally again and inflamed skin breakouts, along with fatigue, disappeared.

Riding the Blood-Sugar Roller Coaster

The primitive part of our brain that's responsible for numerous bodily processes we're not consciously aware of (such as breathing during sleep, blinking when eyes need lubrication) is naturally drawn toward sugar and fat. Thousands of years ago, fruits weren't as sweet as those we find today because they weren't as hybridized to accentuate that taste, and today's refined sugar is concentrated to the point of making our brains go berserk. As expected, eating sugar-laden foods and refined-flour products creates blood-sugar spikes. Unfortunately, these are followed by rapid drops, which makes us hungry for more processed foods. Sound familiar?

High blood-sugar levels can lead to insulin resistance. In turn, this can lead to obesity, high blood pressure, elevated blood fats, and an increased risk of type 2 diabetes because cells are unable to adequately take in sugar.[11] Rebound hypoglycemia (alternating high and low blood sugar) causes mood swings and leads to highs and lows in our thinking, which make us feel as if we're riding an emotional roller coaster.

Processed foods further cause a cascade of problems by stimulating the body's inflammatory response and impeding nitric oxide (which helps dilate arteries and increases blood flow). The B vitamins, particularly important in regulating brain and neurological functioning, are demolished by consuming processed sugar. When B-vitamin levels decrease, cognitive functioning suffers; and we become depressed, angry, anxious, and agitated. Homocysteine levels increase, which make us more susceptible to heart disease and Alzheimer's disease.

The mineral chromium is also negatively affected by processed sugar. Since chromium is a cofactor (helper) in working with insulin, a deficiency causes the sugar to "float" in the bloodstream, exacerbating free-radical activity. This may harm arteries and lead to heart disease. Magnesium is similarly affected, which can lead to a host of problems since it contributes to more than 300 bodily functions. One of the first signs of nutritional deficiencies is altered moods and behavior[12] and it doesn't take a rocket scientist to figure out why these maladies are commonly suffered by kids and many adults today.

Eating whole foods such as oatmeal and brown rice is like placing logs on a fire: They burn slowly, releasing energy over a number of hours. However, when refined flour is consumed (bagels, donuts, cookies, cakes, and the like), it's similar to throwing a piece of paper on a fire—poof! We get an immediate high, soon followed by a low.

Fiber is crucial for helping to regulate blood sugar and fat levels. When we eat grains in their original whole form, the starch is digested slowly because they're full of fiber. The grinding of grains into flour by factory machines increases the grains' surface area—we're essentially having the machines chew our food for us—which allows it to turn into sugar much faster in the body.[13] Refined products affect us similar to injections of sugar directly into an artery. Constant highs and lows leave us wired and tired, ensuring we keep reaching for processed foods over and over. In the coming chapters, you'll learn how to break this cycle.

Legal Drugs?

Did you ever find it difficult to walk past your favorite cookies at the grocery store? That's because even the *thought* of eating certain processed foods stimulates the dopamine pathways in your brain. Refined sugar triggers natural opiates in the brain, similar to narcotics like morphine and heroin,[14] and adding fat (usually in the form of hydrogenated oils) to the mixture multiplies the effect.[15] Since chemically altered foods contribute to unclear thought processes, it's common to start to acting like a drug addict who will do anything to get the next high.

How many of us are using processed foods to self-medicate, numb our feelings, and distract ourselves from the reality of life? Presently, engineered foods have become socially acceptable, legal drugs. When we're euphoric or depressed, we don't celebrate or console ourselves with a plate of broccoli or a raw salad because they don't give us the same high as a sugar cookie or a bowl of ice cream. Natural, wholesome dishes don't allow us to medicate to the same levels as processed foods.

Manufacturers specifically formulate and combine ingredients that will trigger a bigger high in our brain. When we remove processed foods from our diet, we often suffer withdrawal symptoms and cravings. Are processed foods really legal drugs? You decide. Like many drugs, processed foods:

- Reduce immune function
- Deplete the body of nutrients
- Cause cravings and discomfort when eliminated

- Decrease brain function
- Contribute to attention deficit and hyperactivity
- Cause constipation
- Promote dehydration and fatigue
- Contribute to weight gain
- Exacerbate inflammation
- Subsidize company executives with lap-of-luxury living

In all the years that I've worked with food addicts, alcoholics, and drug abusers, no one has ever succeeded when they based their diet on animal products and processed foods. It's common to trade one addiction for another. If someone gives up heroin but trades it for eating processed sugar, they're continuing a cycle of addiction with another modality. The key to real freedom is to stop addictions, in all forms, from stealing their lives. They then gain the ability to fully control their destiny.

Scary Dairy

It's interesting that when people think about building strong bones, dairy products often come to mind. The dairy industry has been pouring billions of dollars into persuading us to wear their "bovine secretion" mustaches.

A male cow doesn't drink his mother's milk past infancy. When we drink cows' milk, we not only consume the lactation product of another species, but we continue to slurp it long after we've been weaned. A male moose, with antlers that can weigh over 70 pounds, doesn't drink his mother's milk past infancy.[16] So where does he get the calcium needed to build those heavy antlers (bones)? From eating plant matter.

Calcium is only one of the nutrients our bones need (along with boron, vitamin D, vitamin K, vitamin C, zinc, and more), and nature provides it abundantly in whole plant foods and sunshine.

Plants absorb calcium and other minerals from the soil, and as they grow, the calcium is built into their roots and stems.[17] Humans don't require excessive amounts of this element if we stop "calcium thieves" from robbing us. These bone bandits include phosphoric acid (an additive in sodas and other processed foods), sugar, salt, caffeine, and nicotine. Lack of exercise is also to blame, being a major contributor to osteoporosis.

When we drink the hormonal secretion of a bovine, we consume a *species-specific mammary-gland discharge never intended for humans.* This hormonal cocktail (cows' milk) is designed to take a 65-pound baby calf and turn him into a 700-pound cow in less than one year—quite a feat. One obvious consequence of people guzzling this concoction is rapid fat gain. Dairy products are one of the leading contributors to the obesity epidemic we're experiencing today. The types of proteins, hormones, and antibodies bovine milk contains are best suited for growing a cow, not a human. People are designed to consume their own mother's milk at least until the age of two.

We're now seeing precocious puberty—girls developing dramatically earlier today than in the past (some as young as eight years old). This may be attributed to the hormones in meat and dairy products, both naturally occurring and those chemically created by agribusiness.[18] Companies are designing bovine growth hormones that force a cow to produce thousands of extra pounds of milk per year. As a result, her udders can become so distended that her teats drag on the ground. In factory-farm concrete lots today, that ground is paved with piles of bacteria-laden manure. The fecal matter contaminates her udders and causes infections (mastitis). This is one of the reasons antibiotics have to be routinely administered (80 percent of the antibiotics produced today are fed to cows, pigs, and chickens). We end up consuming sub-therapeutic doses of antibiotics and bovine growth hormones, along with natural cow hormones in every glass of milk.

Most factory-farm animals are being fed genetically modified crops. Unregulated pesticides contaminate the massive amounts of grains these animals ingest. When we drink body fluids from cattle that consume thousands of doses of toxins over their life span, the residue of poison is delivered to us in a *concentrated* form.

One lethal consequence of consuming dairy products is exposure to insulin-like growth factor 1 (IGF-1), which causes cells to hyper-proliferate. When the dairy industry states that milk builds muscles and bones they fail to disclose that it also *indiscriminately* builds other cells in the body. If we take prostate cancer cells or breast cancer cells and expose them to IGF-1, they grow like weeds, causing disease at an alarming rate.[19] Every sip of milk and every bite of cheese contains IGF-1. Increasing the most powerful hormone in the human body through our diet consumption has effects, many of which are negative and dangerous.[20]

When we're infants, we secrete an enzyme called lactase to digest the sugar lactose in human milk. As we get older, after about the age of two, we gradually slow the secretion of this enzyme and become inefficient at digesting lactose (found in milk). This is one of the reasons many adults are unable to properly digest dairy products and suffer from flatulence, bloating, and stomach upset. Milk allergies are common in kids and frequently cause respiratory, gastrointestinal, and skin problems, along with childhood ear infections.[21]

Casein is a protein found in cow's milk. In his revolutionary book *The China Study,* T. Colin Campbell, Ph.D., showed that in a laboratory setting, they were able to turn cancer "on" and "off" by the amount of casein in the diet.[22] Cheese contains more casein than other dairy products because when milk is turned into cheese, most of its water, whey proteins, and lactose sugar are removed, which leaves behind concentrated casein and fat.

Dairy products are notoriously high in fat. When we see the "2 percent" label prominently displayed on milk cartons, we're under the false impression that the product contains only 2 percent fat. This is not the case. The amount listed is calculated by *volume,* not caloric content. This product derives a whopping 35 percent of its calories from fat. That's quite significant. Is it any wonder that consuming even reduced-fat dairy products increases our chances of obesity? It's now common for me to see new clients walking in the door weighing 350 pounds or more, with young children topping 200 pounds. Dairy products are one of the reasons.

The dairy industry has long sung the benefits of ingesting these products for strong bones and osteoporosis prevention. Their magical, mystical claim to fame is calcium. Because dairy contains this mineral, we're told repeatedly that we must consume it or face negative health consequences. Clinical research has refuted these claims and numerous studies show that these products serve little to no benefit in improving our bones.[23] Furthermore, increased ingestion of dairy products was shown to double the risk of stress fractures.[24] What has displayed a major influence in decreasing our chances of osteoporosis? Exercise![25] Thankfully, we can put our calcium anxiety to rest and trust plants to fulfill our calcium needs.

Processed Foods Spin the Diet Cycle

Today more than ever, many people are trying to reduce anxiety and confusion and anesthetize emotions because of a lost spiritual connection to the earth, each other, and ultimately themselves. We're not devoting much energy to activities that are conducive to introspection, and a great deal of our time is spent on distractions such as overstimulating entertainment, excessive material possessions, and of course, processed foods.

When our moods become unstable, processed foods are the easiest and cheapest legal drugs. Many people eat even when they're not hungry because of boredom, grief, emptiness, loneliness, or rejection. Continuing to stuff ourselves with these calorically high, nutritionally barren "foods" leads to eventual increases in pounds on the scale, inches on the waistline, and plaque in the arteries; and it invites disease.

When we deprive ourselves of sufficient nourishment, we begin to experience emotional imbalances. Feeling emotionally imbalanced or irritated from low blood sugar encourages us to turn away from these uncomfortable moods by reaching for more processed foods as calming, soothing medication. Enter the diet cycle, which can continue for years as we seesaw erratically between gaining and losing weight.

The Diet Cycle

Whole-food, calorie, and nutrient deprivation (diet)
→ emotional imbalance
Emotional imbalance = feelings of regret, irritability,
anger, and frustration
Uncomfortable moods → cravings for processed
foods as calming, soothing medication

Diets are unsuccessful in the long term because they don't address the human being as a whole entity and are not lifestyle habits. Most work well for reducing weight in the short term, but unfortunately they create a disease cycle (heart disease, diabetes, metabolic syndrome, adrenal fatigue, and more) in the body. Dieting does not change our brain chemistry in a positive way or enlighten us about the reasons we were initially overeating.

To experience exuberant energy and a peaceful, balanced mind, we must modify and change our eating habits. The information in the coming chapters will show you how.

CHAPTER 2

BUILDING HEALTH WITH REAL FOOD

What would we eat if we were stranded on a desert island? We'd eat foods grown from the earth: fruits, vegetables, grains, beans, peas, lentils, nuts, tubers, and seeds. We wouldn't consume processed foods because the machinery required to refine them would not be available. The question really comes down to: Could we live a healthy, happy life if we just ate what grew from the earth? The resounding answer is *yes!*

From the beginning of time, *all* people ate foods that grew from the soil. It wasn't until the recent creations of mechanical equipment and synthetic chemicals that we became inundated with cheap processed options. Civilizations have been leading healthy lives for thousands of years by consuming whole foods.

Nature makes it easy for us to eat and has supplied us with an abundance of satisfying, easy to prepare, delicious choices. Today, more than ever, good nutrition is not a luxury—it's a necessity. Preventive medicine is pennies on the dollar compared to our financially draining health-care system. Our need for the protective components found in fruits and vegetables has never been greater.

Magical Warehouses

A diet based on vibrant plant foods is the best lifestyle choice for great health and ensuring the sustainability of our planet. We can take advantage of nature's symphony of nutrients and phytochemicals; they nourish and protect us.

Plants are subjected to ultraviolet sun exposure for numerous hours every day. In addition, they are attacked by fungus and bugs intent on devouring them. Since flora can't run or walk away from threats like humans and animals can, plants have to continually modify their methods of self-defense to stay alive. Their bodies become natural phytoceutical (plant-based remedy) stores that contain antioxidants, vitamins, and minerals, which are used to protect them against outside threats.

When we consume plant matter, we ingest these crucial elements, which in turn help *our* bodies ward off environmental and chemical attacks.[1] This is one of the reasons why foods are so much more than just an entertaining diversion to be used for taste or false mood modification. What we eat contains the potential and power to create either disharmony and disease or health and vibrancy. Hippocrates, the father of modern medicine said, "Let food be thy medicine and medicine be thy food." Plants contain active substances that have tremendous healing properties.[2]

Calorically speaking, plant foods are the most nutrient dense. So why don't we consume more of them? To most people, a salad will never be as attractive as a cookie, but it's important to think of the nutrients delivered, not the entertainment or "high" we may experience.

It's difficult to get too many calories when we eat vast amounts of plant matter because the fiber in plants generates the feeling of fullness before the consumption of too many calories. As we discussed, fiber helps keep blood sugar in a normal range and enhances satiety (the feeling of fullness and satisfaction). It also binds with unwanted, carcinogenic xenoestrogens and other toxic substances and eliminates them from the body, helping prevent their reabsorption.

We all want to eat with feelings of abundance, not deprivation, and plant foods lead the way while sustaining us for a lifetime.

Trust Plant Protein

When people are asked what protein is for, most don't have any idea at all. They simply repeat what they've heard: "We need protein, and lots of it!" Throughout life, this is the jingle we hear from well-funded animal-agribusiness marketing teams and the industries that profit from them. Who asks, "Where do we get our nutrients?" Where is the concern for boron, selenium, chromium, lutein, folate, and lycopene? We're far more deficient in these than we'll ever be in protein.

Protein is important for building and repairing muscle tissue, and it's an integral component of our hair, nails, bone, neurotransmitters, and internal organs. It helps with enzymes, antibodies, and hormones. We don't require much, though, especially after childhood. If we eat an adequate amount of a variety of whole foods, we will receive more than enough, since it's found in all plant foods.[3] Protein is composed of amino acids, which serve as its building blocks similar to the way letters form a word. Our body doesn't care what foods the amino acids come from, as long as we're receiving the required ones in sufficient quantities.

The strongest and largest animals on the planet are herbivores that obtain their protein from plant matter. Gorillas don't eat other animals, yet they're considerably stronger and larger than humans. Shouldn't their needs be greater since they're bigger and more muscular? Large, plant-eating animals (such as rhinoceroses, elephants, giraffes, hippopotamuses, and cows) eat vegetation exclusively. Plant matter supplies all the amino acids their bodies require to create protein.

One analogy I use often with clients is visualizing food as a "container." Animal-flesh containers include a cesspool of antibiotics, hormones, cholesterol, saturated fat, and pesticides—much more than we bargained for in our quest to obtain the almighty protein.[4] This leads us to consume all the nasties we don't want. When we eat plant-based protein, the container is fiber, protein, phytochemicals, and supernutrients—everything we want to preserve our tissues and keep us vibrant.

There's no need to have a protein phobia or specifically combine certain foods at the same meal. Just eat an adequate supply of fruits, vegetables, whole grains, and tubers, and plenty of legumes, along with small amounts of nuts and seeds, and leave the protein fears behind forever.

Good, Better, and Best

Too many people today view life situations as either black or white, good or bad, right or wrong. However, there are many possibilities. Ideally, of course, we want to eat the best foods possible, but sometimes we can't due to reasons beyond our control. This often causes apprehension and worry over not getting the perfect meals for a particular day. Maybe they were good, but we didn't get the best. This is fine because it gives us something to work on tomorrow.

There are different degrees of good, better, and best, and the goal is to always *have the best option.* We do the best we can and should look for progress—not perfection. The key is not to fret over less-than-optimal choices and instead to continually get better and better. If we stress too much over the ideal, it causes more harm than good to the body, mind, and psyche. The key is to focus on improving all the time.

These principles of good, better, and best have worked wonders for my clients. When they release the idea that there's no bad or wrong way to do things, they improve. For example, let's look at an opportunity to squeeze a salad into our day. If we start with some greens and tomatoes, that would be good. Contributing a red bell pepper and some asparagus to the base would be even better. Adding beans and sweet potatoes would be the best because now we'd have a tremendous amount of volume and nutrients in one meal.

Any effort to add whole, unprocessed foods is great and worthy of recognition since they add up in micronutrient content. The secret is to make sure to consume items with the most nutritional benefits first: legumes, green salads, green vegetables, sweet potatoes, and fruits. This leaves limited space for less-than-ideal foods, rather than the other way around.

What would be more filling: a fruit salad made with a chopped apple and two chopped plums, a medium-size cooked yam topped with cinnamon, a pound and a half of broccoli topped with hummus and salsa, or two tablespoons of olive oil? The olive oil has the most calories but takes up the least room in the stomach and has the fewest nutrients. This is why we can consume a quarter cup of oil per day without even being aware of it. However, our *waistlines* will be more than aware and will respond accordingly by expanding from the unused, empty calories.

Vegetables, fruits, legumes, and whole grains are the solid building materials that help hold up our body's foundation. Nutritionally, they give us the most value per calorie. By contrast, refined grains, oils, and processed sugar supply us with little value. The following recommendations have allowed my clients to solidly build an enjoyable eating plan. Use them to help guide you in the right direction of building a solid pillar of health.

Take a look at the following chart:

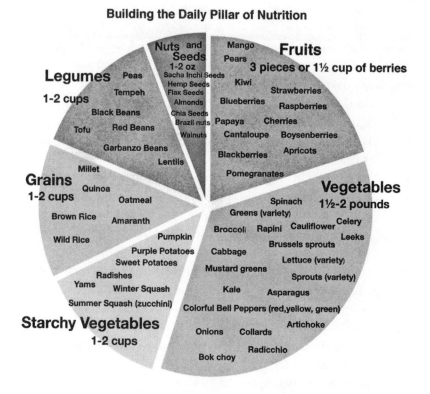

Building the Daily Pillar of Nutrition

It's a good starting point to keep in mind when looking at the daily meal menu. The volume of food will depend greatly on your physical activity and individual needs. The key is to focus on the *quality* of the food.

Vegetables should make up a good part of our diet (particularly green leafy vegetables), followed by fruits (with a large emphasis on a variety of berries), legumes, whole grains, starchy vegetables, and a small amount of nuts and seeds. The following foods are shown in the chart in order of significance.

— **Green leafy vegetables:** These are the most important power foods we can ingest. Green leafy vegetables contain, ounce for ounce, the most nutrients, phytochemicals, vitamins, and minerals. While the lowest in calories, they still provide the necessary fats and protein we need for optimal nutrition. Some examples include kale; collards; turnip greens; spinach; mustard greens; Swiss chard; red, green, and romaine lettuce; arugula; and dandelion greens. Most of my clients eat these without restriction.

— **Cruciferous vegetables:** These contain some of the highest anticancer properties known. Be sure to chew or blend these vegetables very well to release and enhance the preventive substances found inside. Some examples are broccoli, cabbage, cauliflower, brussels sprouts, bok choy, rapini (broccoli rabe), Chinese or napa cabbage, rutabaga, radishes, and daikon.

— **Fruits:** Naturally sweet and universally appealing, fruits offer a tremendous variety of delicious goodness. Enjoy at least three pieces per day or 1½ cups of berries. Explore unusual options like mango and kiwi rather than the common apples, oranges, and bananas. Focus on berries such as boysenberries, blueberries, raspberries, and strawberries. Pomegranates are also a great choice.

— **Legumes:** Protein-rich beans, peas, and lentils are also high in lysine, an important amino acid that we need daily for optimal health. The resistant starches found in beans make them less calorically available than other foods, which means that we can enjoy them in greater quantities. They're one of the best sources of fiber, which helps to regulate blood sugar and cholesterol. Satisfying and filling, legumes are a wonderful way to get B vitamins and protein. Foods in this category include adzuki beans, black beans, garbanzo beans, kidney beans, pinto beans, soybeans, green peas, and lentils. My clients have found success with eating 1 to 2 cups of legumes per day.

— **Whole grains:** Consuming about 1 to 2 cups of whole grains a day has benefited many of my clients. Slow-cooked oatmeal (not instant), quinoa, millet, amaranth, and brown rice are filling and nutritious, providing fiber, vitamins, minerals, antioxidants, and healthy fats. Those who are watching their caloric load can consume 1/2 cup per day or none at all.

— **Starchy vegetables:** Potatoes are universally enjoyed and are some of the most filling and satisfying foods. I recommend that sweet potatoes, yams, and purple potatoes make up the menu plan when choosing from this group. Colorful varieties contain substantially more phytochemicals and should account for most of our consumption. Purple potatoes have been shown to decrease inflammation in the body[5] and should be sought out when looking to include potatoes in the diet. Other starchy vegetables include summer squash, winter squash, pumpkin, and radishes.

— **Nuts:** I recommend eating nuts sparingly, particularly if weight gain, cardiovascular issues, or diabetes is a concern. Between one and two ounces daily or less is sufficient for most people (choose from nuts or seeds). I suggest sprinkling a few on salads or incorporating them into a smoothie recipe. It's easy to lose control when eating nuts from bags and boxes, as we tend to eat them by the handful, especially if they're roasted in oil and have added sugar and salt. Nuts are valuable for their phytosterol content, which may help reduce cholesterol. Nuts contain vitamins (particularly the important antioxidant vitamin E, severely lacking in most people's diets), minerals, and protein. Consider choosing Brazil nuts, walnuts, almonds, pecans, and pistachios.

— **Seeds:** These are rich in protein, minerals, B vitamins, fat, and dietary fiber. Alternate eating nuts and seeds on different days if possible, consuming about an ounce or two daily. Simply sprinkle a few teaspoons on top of a salad, in smoothies, or in oatmeal, or incorporate them into main dishes. Flaxseeds should always be ground and placed in the refrigerator for storage. Good options include sunflower seeds, pumpkin seeds, flaxseeds, hemp seeds, chia seeds, and sacha inchi seeds.

Fueling Up on Smoothies

Ah . . . the joy of smoothies. Just the name invokes pleasant images of our day becoming happier and smoother. When we blend fruits and vegetables, we break down their fibers and help release their nutrients. Since many of us don't chew our food thoroughly enough, drinking high-nutrient, raw, whole foods allows us to digest and assimilate larger volumes of plants. Smoothies provide the perfect quick pick-me-up and are a great way to incorporate several servings of fruits or vegetables into our day.

I encourage smoothies for other reasons, too: First, children don't eat enough plant matter, which makes blended liquids a fair, logical, and healthy alternative. When we place six to seven types of fruits or vegetables into a morning smoothie, kids are able to drink it without much fuss. If they were asked to eat a bowl of spinach, blueberries, mangos, and green beans, the chances of that happening for breakfast would be quite slim. Often, many kids run out the door in the morning after ingesting a "sugar feast" of processed foods, or they skip eating altogether. Drinking a smoothie provides a flavorful and nutritious solution. Would it be better if kids ate six or seven bowls of fruits and vegetables per day? Of course! But until they do, a tasty smoothie is a doable alternative. Second, smoothies are a blessing to seniors who chew poorly. Much of our elderly population suffers from impaired digestion (hydrochloric acid and digestive enzymes are low), and psychologically it's difficult for them to handle eating large volumes of plant matter. Putting whole fruits and vegetables into a smoothie lets them maximize the nutrients they ingest and enjoy a wonderful elixir that's lifesaving to them.

Over the course of my more than two decades working with hard-core athletes, I have seen how smoothies play a crucial role in enhancing sports performance and recovery. When these individuals work out extremely hard, they have a tendency to lose their appetite immediately afterward. Since they don't feel hungry, they often stop eating and fail to consume the nutrients needed for recuperation. One thing they're willing to do is drink. By ingesting a smoothie, they maximize their nutrition without being overwhelmed by food volume. This also helps save digestive energy (necessary for recovery) and prevents additional fatigue.

The versatility and portability of smoothies make them fast and convenient. The sky is the limit since we can blend every healthy combination under the sun. Investing in a good blender with a powerful motor (my clients enjoy Blendtec) will make for easier mixing and provide a creamier texture. Older blenders without much power get stuck more often and place greater stress on the motor, leading to breakage. To lessen the load, make smaller batches, stir often, and add ingredients slowly.

Make sure to use fresh or frozen organic fruits and vegetables, not canned (except for pumpkin). Soaking dried fruit and using both the fruit and water will add a nutrient-rich base. Dehydrated fruit that hasn't been soaked in advance will be too hard and won't blend as well. The exceptions are dates, figs, and raisins, which can be added in small amounts for sweetness, nutrients, and fiber.

The few occasions when I don't recommend smoothies high in fruit are when clients seek weight loss or suffer from diabetes or cardiovascular disease. In some cases, I may suggest that 70 to 80 percent of a smoothie be composed of green vegetables, with only a small portion containing berries.

Always keep frozen fruits and vegetables available because it's easy to place them in the blender with nut milk, coconut water, or just plain water. They can be prepared almost instantly. Be sure to make extra in the morning, pour some in an airtight container, place in the freezer for 20 minutes, and then take it on the go to sip throughout the day.

Enjoy the following recipes or create your own!

PUMPKIN PIE SMOOTHIE

¼ cup cooked pumpkin or ¼ can organic pumpkin puree
4 cups almond milk (fresh or packaged)
1 cup blueberries (fresh or frozen)
3–4 dates (pitted)
2 chard leaves or 2 cups greens of choice
1 ripe pear (cored)

Mix all ingredients in a blender.

Makes 2–3 servings

(Feel free to add a plant-based protein powder to your smoothie as desired. My clients enjoy the Boku, Sunwarrior, Vega, and Warrior Force brands.)

PURPLE POWER SMOOTHIE

3 cups coconut water
1–3 leaves of purple kale or 2 cups greens of choice
3 dates (pitted)
1 apple (cored)
1 cup blueberries
2 tbsp raisins

Mix all the ingredients well in a blender and enjoy.

Makes 2–3 servings.

(Try adding green powders to your smoothies for an additional nutritional boost. My clients enjoy the Vitamineral Green powder from HealthForce Nutritionals and the Super Food powder from Boku.)

Buy Any Greens Necessary

Greens play a critical role in our diet because they provide us with vitamins, minerals, and phytonutrients. Unfortunately, the majority of people aren't eating nearly enough of them, for a variety of reasons. Some people don't enjoy the taste of greens while others mistakenly believe that only a few leaves on a sandwich are sufficient. Those suffering from intestinal problems or digestive issues find large volumes of greens difficult to "stomach" and consequently end up avoiding them altogether. People with limited grocery-shopping schedules often find they run out of greens well before their next trip to the store and miss out on eating any in the interim. All of these impediments make it challenging to get enough greens, and as a result, many fail to consume one of the most important components of green vegetables: chlorophyll.

Chlorophyll is one of the key essential elements found in greens. It's a plant pigment that gives green vegetables their vibrant green color. Chlorophyll has been known to bind to carcinogens and toxins, preventing them from causing cellular damage. With the continual bombardment of toxic substances in our environment, we need chlorophyll's help now more than ever before.

Additionally, the fruits and vegetables our grandparents enjoyed in their youth were more abundant in vitamins and minerals than many varieties we have access to today. Modern intensive agriculture methods have stripped increasing amounts of nutrients from the earth and left us with a disturbing trend of soil depletion. Since plants absorb nutrients found in the ground, the poorer their growth environment, the lower their nutritional content. Harvesting, packaging, transporting, and extended time on the shelf further diminishes their nutritional value.

This is the reason I advocate the use of concentrated, quality, green drinks as a means of "bathing" the cells with more magnified nutrients. Green powders and juices can provide detoxifying and alkalinizing support we could all use more of. Adding green powders to clean water or smoothies becomes an easy way to incorporate concentrated nutrition into our diet.

There are many types of green powders on the market today. Some contain single ingredients such as wheatgrass or barley grass, but many others consist of combinations of greens, such as grasses, herbs, vegetable and fruit extracts, sprouted legumes, and algae. This increases their nutritional benefits and ensures that we ingest more vitamins, minerals, enzymes, chlorophyll, and phytonutrients—a multitude of essential nutrients we need to optimize our health.

While green powders can help supplement our needs, this doesn't mean that we shouldn't make a diligent effort to consume sufficient amounts of fresh fruits and green vegetables—we should. But if our greens consumption is low or nonexistent, and circumstances don't allow a shift to a greater volume of fresh greens, these products can help bridge the gap.

Since many of us have access to clean water during the day, why not maximize every sip by adding a teaspoon of green powder to it? This way you're continually bathing your cells with antioxidants and chlorophyll. My clients have experienced very successful results by taking a water container mixed with one tablespoon of a green powder such as Vitamineral Green from HealthForce Nutritionals for sipping throughout the day.

Monumental Salads

Crisp, colorful, nutritious, and delicious, salads are attractive and appealing. One pound of green leafy vegetables contains only 125 calories, so we don't have to feel guilty about filling up on these low-calorie, nutrient-packed foods at the beginning of every meal.

If you wish to add a dressing to make the salad even more enjoyable, make sure it contributes additional nutrients. The blender is a great tool to use for making fresh, appetizing salad dressings. Adding a red bell pepper to some avocado and fresh carrot juice in a blender will result in a mouthwatering, creamy mixture. Pouring this delightful treat over fresh vegetables makes eating even more enjoyable and nourishing. Try adding fresh or dried herbs such as oregano or basil, or some garlic, for a zestier treat. Other nutrient-packed toppings include salsa, guacamole, hummus, baba ghanoush, and tahini (ground sesame seeds). Experiment with tossing in raisins, dried cranberries, chopped apricots, or nuts and seeds (in small amounts) for additional texture and flavor. The fat in nuts, seeds, and avocados helps us absorb the nutrients in the salad.

I recommend that meals be primarily centered on generous-size salads. These should always be consumed first, regardless of what is eaten afterward. My clients have found this to be effective because it allows them to consume abundant amounts of plant matter, and they feel delightfully satisfied. Remember, a salad isn't just lettuce. It may include sweet potatoes, beans, a variety of steamed vegetables, and a nutrient-filled dressing along with green leafy vegetables.

Crunching and chewing is important because it allows us to release the vegetables' nutrients. Chewing thoroughly helps relieve tension in the jaw, a common place where we hold stress. Taking the time to eat slowly, with reverence, assists us in enjoying and appreciating the food. Our brain also gets the signal that we're eating a meal, which makes us feel fuller faster. A complete salad is filled with plant matter that's packed with fiber and nutrients. It's low in fat and has no cholesterol—a perfect meal.

Salads don't have to be cold, and the flavors can be enhanced with heated or warmed vegetables. Experiment with toppings of mashed sweet potatoes or freshly steamed vegetables and allow them to sit for a few minutes to gently heat the ingredients underneath.

Try the following salads and homemade dressings or invent new creations that delight the taste buds. Be sure to share your inspiring combinations with family and friends.

VISUAL MASTERPIECE SALAD WITH DRESSING

2 cups salad greens
½ red bell pepper (sliced)
½ yellow bell pepper (sliced)
1 tomato (sliced)
½ cup cucumber (sliced)
½ cup garbanzo beans (cooked)
1 tbsp pine nuts or walnuts

Dressing
1 tbsp tahini (ground sesame seeds)
¼ cup carrot juice
⅛ tsp onion powder
dash of your favorite spices (such as dill, cilantro, basil, or oregano)

Mix dressing ingredients in a blender until creamy.
Pour over salad. Toss and enjoy!

Makes 1–2 servings.

ARUGULA SWEET-AND-SPICY SALAD WITH DRESSING

2 cups arugula
1 tbsp dried cranberries
2 tbsp raw walnut pieces
1 cup sprouts of choice
1 cup sweet potato (steamed and sliced)

Dressing
3 small tangerines (peeled)
1 tsp miso paste (white mellow miso)
2 dates (pitted)
dash of cayenne pepper (optional)

Combine dressing ingredients in a blender until creamy.
Pour over salad and toss well. Serve immediately. Enjoy!

Makes 1–2 servings.

CUCUMBER-MINT SALAD

1 large cucumber (finely sliced)
5–7 mint leaves (minced)
½ avocado (mashed)
1 tsp dill powder
⅛ tsp cayenne powder (optional)
2 tbsp pine nuts (optional)
dash of your favorite spices (such as cilantro, ginger, turmeric, or oregano)

Combine all ingredients in a bowl. Mix well. Use as a salad or a side dish to a main meal.

Makes 1–2 servings.

What's More Filling and Nutritious?

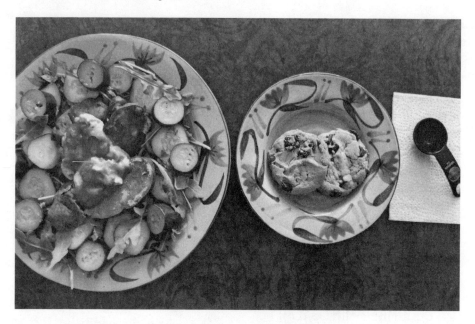

This photo displays a plate of salad, a plate of two cookies, and a tablespoon of olive oil. Which plate would satiate hunger and provide the most nutrients? The ingredients, calories, and notable nutrients are found below.

Salad Ingredients

2 cups arugula
Total calories: 10
Fat: 0 g
Sugar: 1 g
Protein: 1 g

Notable nutrients: Vitamin K: 43 mcg, Calcium: 64 mg, Magnesium: 19 mg

Source: USDA National Database for Standard Reference, http://ndb.nal
.usda.gov/

1 cup tomato
Total calories: 21
Fat: 0 g
Sugar: 0 g
Protein: 1 g

Notable nutrients: Potassium: 359 mg, Folate: 42 mcg, Vitamin C: 12.5 mg

Source: USDA National Database for Standard Reference, http://ndb.nal
.usda.gov/

½ cup cucumber
Total calories: 8
Fat: 0 g
Sugar: 1 g
Protein: .34 g

Notable nutrients: Calcium: 8 mg, Phosphorus: 12 mg, Potassium: 76 mg

Source: USDA National Database for Standard Reference, http://ndb.nal
.usda.gov/

Steamed purple potatoes (3 small)
Total calories: 165
Fat: 0 g
Sugar: 0 g
Protein: 5 g

Notable nutrients: Calcium: 703 mg, high content of anthocyanin (purple
pigment), which may supply anti-inflammatory properties to our body[6]

Source: Calorie Gallery, Purple Potatoes, http://www.caloriegallery.com
/foods/calories-in-purple-potatoes.htm

1 medium zucchini (steamed)
Total calories: 33
Fat: 1 g
Sugar: 5 g
Protein: 2 g

Notable nutrients: Potassium: 512 mg, Calcium: 31 mg, Vitamin A: 392 IU

Source: USDA National Database for Standard Reference, http://ndb.nal
.usda.gov/

2 tbsp oil-free hummus
Total calories: 35
Fat: 2 g
Sugar: 0 g
Protein: 2 g

Be sure to buy hummus without added oil. It makes a wonderful creamy
dressing alone or when paired with salsa.

Source: http://www.livestrong.com/thedailyplate/nutrition-calories/food
/trader-joes/eggplant-hummus/

2 tbsp oil-free salsa
Total calories: 10

It has a nominal nutritional profile, but salsa adds a zesty taste to salads,
which makes the dish more appealing and appetizing.

Source: http://www.livestrong.com/thedailyplate/nutrition-calories
/food/trader-joes/organic-salsa/

Total calories for the salad: 282

2 chocolate-chip cookies
Total calories: 420
Fat: 22 g
Sugar: 32 g
Protein: 3 g

Nutrient content: nominal

Source: SparkPeople. "Calories in Costco Chocolate Chip Cookie,"
http://www.sparkpeople.com/calories-in.asp?food=costco+chocolate+
chip+cookie

1 tbsp olive oil
Total calories: 119
Fat: 14 g
Sugar: 0 g
Protein: 0 g

Nutrient content: nominal

Source: USDA National Database for Standard Reference, http://ndb.nal
.usda.gov/

What would happen if we poured the tablespoon of olive oil on top of the salad and ate the cookies for dessert? Our consumption would go from 282 calories and 3 grams of fat to 821 calories and 39 grams of fat in just one meal!

CHAPTER 3

BRINGING IT ALL TOGETHER

I'm frequently asked what people should eat, and the answer is always different because each individual is unique. It's difficult to recommend the same menu plan for everyone because we all have distinctive tastes, preferences, and needs. Sedentary individuals have different caloric requirements from athletes and growing children need nutritional support that varies from seniors. But while the quantities of food consumed may change, the base makeup of the whole foods will remain virtually the same. It's similar to asking how many plates to bring to a party: It depends on how many people will be attending. The one thing that won't change is that plates will be needed and used. Remember, when you choose whole foods, you help re-sensitize your taste buds and nutritious ingredients start to taste better than ever.

Simple Meals to Build On

I created a few basic menu ideas that many of my clients find appetizing, nourishing, filling, and cost effective. I specifically chose whole foods that are readily available just about everywhere.

Breakfast Ideas

- Slow-cooked oatmeal (not instant) with blueberries, walnuts or ground flaxseeds, almond milk, and a sprinkle of cinnamon
- Smoothie with generous amounts of greens and berries or other fruit
- Tofu sautéed in water (not oil) with seasoning such as turmeric and garlic, served with raw or steamed vegetables

Lunch Ideas

- Large salad with greens, raw vegetables of choice, and cooked beans
- Sandwich wrap, using chard leaves or brown-rice tortillas, filled with sprouts, hummus, cucumbers, tomatoes, avocado, and red bell peppers
- Veggie and bean soup with your favorite vegetables and purple potatoes

Dinner Ideas

- Chard or collard greens with sweet potatoes or purple potatoes and black-bean salsa
- Brown rice with assorted vegetables and tempeh
- Quinoa with steamed cauliflower and green beans
- Spinach soup with assorted vegetables and beans
- Variety of steamed squash with lentils, avocado, and steamed garlic

Snack Ideas

- Celery, carrots, and zucchini sticks with hummus, salsa, or guacamole

- Handful of raw walnuts, raw almonds, or Brazil nuts

- Blackberries, blueberries, raspberries, or strawberries with dairy-free cultured coconut milk (my clients enjoy the So Delicious brand)

Tips to Implement Today

- Purge your kitchen of processed foods and commit to not buying them anymore. When your home is free of unhealthy options, it's harder to revert to old habits. Put all processed foods in bags or boxes and give them away to a food pantry.

- If you're worried that fresh vegetables will spoil, it's perfectly fine to buy frozen, since they're frequently frozen the same day they're picked.

- Keep healthy snacks in your car, purse, or travel bag. Good choices are fresh fruit, trail mix, raw almonds, raw sunflower or pumpkin seeds, or food bars (Organic Food Bars, Evo Hemp, Boku Bars, and Journey Bar brands).

- Read ingredient labels. Avoid foods containing unhealthy fats (hydrogenated fats) or sweeteners (refined sugar) or unrecognizable ingredients.

- Pick a day to shop for vegetables. Wash, chop, and store them in glass or stainless-steel containers for the upcoming week. When you open the refrigerator door and have a colorful cornucopia of vegetables, washed, prepped, and ready to go, it becomes easy to make a quick salad in a large bowl.

- Cook beans, grains, and oatmeal in sizable quantities in advance and store them in the freezer or fridge for quick reheating.

- Buy organic, local, and fair-trade produce. This supports local farmers and their families.

- Eat moderate amounts and in a relaxed manner.

- Buy in bulk to reduce packaging and waste. (It's also cheaper.)

- Bring a bag to the store when shopping to reduce waste.

- Share wholesome foods with your friends and family. Everyone benefits from sampling tasty and nutritious items prepared with love.

Cleaning Up Greasy Plates

Are you experiencing an oil slick on your plate? You may be if you're indiscriminately pouring on lots of oil, assuming it's a health food.

There's no refined oil found in nature—this is a clue. We come across whole olives, nuts, and avocados but not olive, macadamia, or avocado oil. Similar to processed sugar, oil is an unnatural product and happens to be the most calorie-dense food in the world—a whopping 4,000 calories per pound!

The biggest culprit when it comes to weight gain, lethargy, and blood-sugar problems is the overconsumption of oils, regardless of their source. They turn rancid quickly due to the removal of life-sustaining antioxidants and the caustic refining methods manufacturers use to extract oils from whole foods to make them appear "clear" for aesthetic purposes. They cause premature aging and cellular distortion (due to rancidity), and should be omitted from the diet completely. No one has ever died from an olive-oil deficiency. There's nothing particularly magical about olive oil other than it's a healthier alternative to animal fat.

By nature's design, humans are meant to store fat. This makes perfect sense from a survival standpoint: If there's a famine, we will remain alive. We require a certain amount of fat to procreate and ensure the safety of the next generation. Storing fat is fine as long as it's not out of control. The problem we're having today is that we've far exceeded our limitation and moved into the "fat-osphere." As oil moved into the diet, people became heavier and heavier (our bodies love to store fat).

The body craves fat more than almost anything because this macronutrient is difficult to find in sizable quantities in nature. In the past, we had to compete with animals and climb trees to procure fatty nuts, then work tediously to remove their shells. Instinctively, we didn't gorge on them all at once, but saved them for times of severe famine, knowing they were the perfect food for long-term survival.

All fat is approximately nine calories per gram, and the body stores it all the same. Fats add texture to food, increase satiety, and supply us with essential fatty acids (the building blocks of hormones). We're able to burn fatty acids for fuel.

Most fried foods, processed foods, and animal fats (from dairy products, eggs, and meat) contain saturated fats or trans fats—both of which can contribute to heart disease and other health conditions. Many processed foods contain hidden oils in their ingredients, and all of those fat grams add up.

From a nutritional standpoint, the main reason to eat some whole foods that contain fats is because they help with the absorption of carotenoids and carry fat-soluble vitamins (A, D, K, and E), assisting in their transport around the body. We use essential fatty acids to regulate our immune function, control arterial dilation and inflammation, and promote proper retinal development and optimal neurological functioning. Essential fatty acids can be created in the body by eating nuts, seeds, and green leafy vegetables. Fats also help regulate prostaglandins (hormone-like substances), protect us from injury by cushioning our organs and glands, and provide long-term energy.

I'm fond of recommending nuts and seeds in small quantities because they are a source of minerals, protein, and phytosterols, and they assist in reducing cholesterol. Brazil nuts are especially high in selenium, an important mineral for immune function. Throw some nuts on salads and be sure to buy only the raw, unsalted variety.

If you're used to frying vegetables with oil, try steaming them with water instead. Be sure to keep an eye on the pan, as the water will evaporate much quicker than oil.

Simply eliminating oil has helped numerous people lose unwanted pounds without feeling hungry or deprived. It keeps caloric intake down and allows us to enjoy a greater volume of more nutrient-dense foods.

Harvesting Pristine Foods

There are many challenges facing food growth and production today. Genetically modified foods are a huge concern, as are harmful pesticides and other chemicals sprayed on crops.

One way you can take power back and help transform our world for the better is to start an organic garden in your backyard. If you live in an apartment and have access to a small balcony, you can still make a difference by buying a few containers, seeds, and some organic soil. Some neighborhoods have community gardens that can be joined for free or a nominal fee, and you can always help a friend or neighbor tend their garden if it's impossible to have your own.

Growing vegetables, herbs, and fruits has never been easier. You can even reuse food waste as compost to help nourish your plants. Seeds from vegetables grown this year can be used to plant more the next season. The same pots and tools can be reused over and over. You'll also save on food costs by consuming your harvest and sharing any additional food with family and friends. What could make a better gift to loved ones than fresh, organic produce cultivated with love in your garden?

Growing food is a relaxing, energizing experience that connects us with the earth again—and ultimately with ourselves. Watching plants thrive from our efforts is fulfilling, enjoyable, and recharging. We become more attuned to nature and the cycle of life.

If you can't have soil-filled containers because you live in a small space, you can still reap enormous benefits by sprouting indoors. There are numerous wonderful websites and retailers dedicated to providing easy-to-follow instructions on sprouting from fabric bags, glass jars, and other containers. Sprouts grow quickly, and numerous varieties can be easily cultivated and enjoyed. They make wonderful additions to salads and just about any meal. They're rich in chlorophyll, packed with nutrients, and cheap to grow at home, requiring very little space or investment of time.

Today's kids (and many adults) spend little time actively participating in growing plant foods. If we start teaching children how to garden and sprout, they'll make the much-needed connection about where whole foods come from. Many children are saturated with disguised "foods" in boxes and believe that meals only come from factories or take-out places. When they actively participate and learn about soil, water, sunshine, and individual plant needs, they gain valuable reasons to care about our planet. Gardening offers exercise while teaching useful skills. We can help turn our children into lifelong fruit and vegetable fans if they actively participate in growing their own foods and take pride in the harvest. They're also much more likely to eat the healthy foods they had a hand in growing.

Gardening and sprouting empowers all of us and allows us to maintain direct control over our soil, ensuring that harmful pesticides don't end up in the ground and then in our body. Our gardens can help provide safe havens for wildflowers, insects, small animals, and birds. What could be more beautiful than seeing the dazzling movement of butterflies and bees and hearing birds in the backyard?

The mere sight of a garden helps improve our emotions and sense of well-being. Many gardeners also experience a type of "meditation in motion." These feelings of peace and contentment are cultivated while we enrich and nurture the soil. Planting and deciding on which fruits and veggies we'll grow develops mental creativity that's vital for cognitive function. Gardening also improves hand-eye coordination and stimulates the sense of smell. The list of benefits is seemingly endless.

Saving Whole Foods

It's sobering to think that those of us born before the mass adulteration of whole foods may be the last generation to have the experience of enjoying how good they are. Will we be the only ones left who can compare what real food was like and what machinery has turned it into—an unrecognizable and dangerous creation?

Are tomorrow's children going to recognize whole foods, or will they only know processed foods? Will they search for what whole foods used to look like online, much like researching ancient ruins? Are the remaining organically grown foods today destined to be the dinosaurs of tomorrow?

If trends continue to escalate toward genetically modified, altered foods, this will be the last generation in the history of humanity to experience whole, unprocessed foods the way nature intended. If we do not insist on organic, nontoxic whole foods, what will our future look like? What future . . . ?

Above All, Make It With Love

Meal preparation and cooking is special in many societies, as it should be. Handling food with feelings of love and gratitude is an essential component in building our pillar of nutrition.

Just about everyone has had the experience of a family member or a loved one making a tasty meal. But then it seems that no matter what we do to duplicate their efforts, the result just tastes different. Chances are that when they're cooking for us, they're doing it with a feeling of love. They want the food to taste good and it usually does. On the other hand, when we make something to eat in a hurry and are feeling sad or angry, it just doesn't taste as delightful.

It's important to slow down and enjoy the process. In our mad-rush existence, we often don't have the time or energy to make this happen. Food is often wolfed down as we run out the door to the next pressing event on the agenda.

Let's focus on making every bite count. Most of us are on automatic pilot when we eat. Stop and smell the food. Soon it will become a part of your hair, nails, brain, muscles, attitude, feelings, and energy. Take a moment to appreciate the process that made the food on your plate possible. Someone planted seeds, watered them, checked on the progress of growth, and picked the ripe pro-duce (often under a hot sun). Later it was transported, unloaded, and placed on display at the store or market where it was bought. Now, with your attention, it sits on your plate, ready to finally be transformed into your being. Send the food and everyone who was instrumental in bringing it to your table a silent thank-you. Feel the gratitude and make loving eye contact with the meal.

Above all, prepare food with love and eat it with appreciation. The difference in taste and enjoyment will become profound and will add to your health and exuberant energy.

Part II

THE PILLAR
OF MIND

CHAPTER 4

CARING FOR
OUR MARBLES

If we were to build a computer the size of the tallest building on earth, it would still fail to match the complexity and diversity of the human brain. This intricate three-pound "universe" gracefully situated on top of our shoulders is the most complex active structure on our planet.

In the context of serving as a pillar, the brain requires extra-special attention and support because this superstructure runs much of the show we call life. If we think of physical structure as a house, our brain is responsible for all the actions that make the house a home. The brain would be the thermostat that regulates the indoor temperature, the alarm system that alerts us to threats, the source of electricity powering all devices, and so much more.

With all the immense, round-the-clock responsibilities and demands placed upon our biological superstructure, it makes sense that we'd take immaculate care of it, but many people hardly give it a thought, choosing instead to take better care of a new car or smartphone than this remarkable work of nature.

Over the past 25 years, I observed a significant shift in the reasons people requested my assistance. Previously, new clients' primary focus centered on weight loss, diet, and fitness; but as the decades passed, they increasingly desired more support for mental concerns. I began to hear new clients state, "I feel like I'm losing my marbles," "I'm going bonkers," "I can't focus anymore," "It's just all too much for me mentally," and "My memory is going downhill." I witnessed my office fill up with individuals who suffered from attention deficit disorder, hyperactivity, and depression. Sadly, growing numbers of concerned parents brought their children, who were exhibiting increased aggression and violence. After analyzing their diet and lifestyle habits, it became crystal clear that processed foods, lack of creative mental stimulation, a sedentary lifestyle, and constant stress had begun to take a negative toll not just on the body, but also on the mind.

The brain intimately controls every second of our existence, but the last time many of us even thought about what's inside our head was in seventh-grade biology class. This never truly gave us the opportunity to learn about the critical importance of our brain. No lectures were provided to educate us in how to keep the brain working at its best, but that's about to change.

By the time you finish reading the chapters in this section, The Pillar of Mind, you'll have the tools and techniques you need to keep your brain functioning at its best. Mental health can be greatly affected through ordinary, accessible means such as healthy foods, powerful herbs and spices, a positive attitude, brain-challenging games, mind-expanding thinking, and, in some cases, the use of supplements. I'll discuss these topics in the following chapters, and you'll acquire the know-how to care for your biological superstructure while gaining a new appreciation for its miraculous functions.

Declining Brain Function

We know that the detrimental Standard American Diet (no longer confined to just the United States) is filled with cheap, chemical-based, taste-enhancing additives and mind-altering combinations of fat, sugar, and salt. Inevitably, these menacing products subject consumers to consistent "brain attacks," harming our biological marvel and accomplishing their sinister work with the expected result of *drastic cognitive decline*.

Diseases such as dementia (Alzheimer's in particular), vascular strokes, and brain trauma (inflicted by physical injury, alcohol, tobacco, animal products, and chemical concoctions in processed food) should serve as sufficient motivation for prompting us to make healthy choices that decrease the chances of these maladies from occurring.

Just as most heart disease is influenced by diet and lifestyle factors, dementia is often caused by dietary and environmentally induced inflammation, along with brain assault from toxic substances such as heavy metals (aluminum, mercury, and more). Lack of oxygen and protective nutrients are also large factors. Studies have shown that the risk of Alzheimer's disease is greater in people who consume diets high in cholesterol and saturated fats, and low in fiber, vegetables, and fruits.[1]

Alzheimer's disease is of particular concern to many people because this loss of brain function affects memory, thinking, language, judgment, behavior, and ultimately all body functions. The resulting reduction in cognitive ability is shattering, both to the person afflicted and, perhaps even more so, to the family members and loved ones who struggle to deal with the emotional, physical, and financial hardship it inflicts. The suffering experienced by loved ones when they attempt to communicate with a family member who no longer recognizes them (or their very own image in the mirror) is almost incomprehensible. It's a devastating disease and all preventive measures should be taken to decrease the likelihood of its manifestation.

My personal hands-on experience in working with individuals who suffer from cognitive challenges shows that diet and lifestyle factors can *greatly* assist in keeping the brain healthy. Cognitive issues can be lessened and often improve significantly with dietary diligence, persistence with stimulating brain activities, time, and most important of all—*love*. Love's tremendous contribution to brain and overall health includes stress reduction; the activation of brain areas responsible for emotion, attention, motivation, and memory; and so much more. Love exerts protective effects on the brain.[2] I'll discuss the significance of love and compassion in greater detail later in the book, but for now, keep love and compassion in "mind" as powerful brain helpers.

Frail Building Materials

I've discussed the detrimental effects processed foods have on our body, but it's especially crucial to understand that these products also lack the ability to supply us with the essential nutrients we desperately need to build our neurotransmitters. These chemical messengers convey information instantly from one nerve to another. Optimal brain functioning is dependent on proper neurotransmitter levels and neglecting them leads us into serious mental trouble.

If our neurotransmitter production is low or imbalanced, we may feel drained, unfocused, and depressed. Additionally, we may experience restless high energy in the evening when going to sleep and feel lethargic in the morning upon waking. Important information that needs to be immediately relayed to and from the brain may be delayed or impeded.

Amino acids (the building blocks of protein) help create neurotransmitters. For example, if our body needs to make serotonin, a feel-good neurotransmitter that infuses us with happiness, it will need the amino acid tryptophan. Converting tryptophan to serotonin requires the assistance of critical vitamins and minerals. If we're lacking in these essential nutrients, the transformation won't take place.

Converting amino acids into neurotransmitters is a *synchronistic process* that calls for a host of symphony players such as vitamin B6, vitamin B12, folate, zinc, magnesium, and more. The B vitamins are of significant importance in brain function because they assist our nervous system. If we're deficient in any one of these critical teammates, how will our body make neurotransmitters?

A diet overflowing with processed foods is an invitation to a nutritional deficiency of critical neurotransmitter collaborators. Not only are we *denied* most of these vitamins and minerals in processed foods, but they harm us by using our body's nutrient reserves. How do they do it? Processed sugar gobbles up our B vitamins, chromium, and magnesium, when the body is forced to use them to convert the sugar to energy.

The average American eats 150 pounds of sugar *every year.* One soda contains eight to nine teaspoons alone. Much of the sugar in processed foods is hidden, and eating at restaurants provides doses of sugar and salt (along with MSG and other flavor enhancers) many of us would frown upon. Since most eating establishments are not required to disclose ingredients, we simply *never know* how much we really consume.

Even if we're getting the amino acids we need from our diet, if we're nutrient deficient, we won't have the necessary players (vitamins and minerals) needed to build our neurotransmitters. Imagine sitting down to listen to a symphony orchestra featuring dozens of musicians. If all the players performed together and everyone did their job, we would enjoy hearing a gloriously beautiful musical arrangement. However, what if only one player showed up while the others were stranded because the bus taking them to the performance never showed up? Would the concert be affected? Absolutely. Our brain experiences a similar impact when the needed players (micronutrients) don't show up in our diet.

Thankfully, we have direct control on influencing and building our neurotransmitters from what we choose to eat. We can leverage our brain health for the better with food. Excellent cognitive function starts in the kitchen because that's where the nutritional materials (whole foods) are prepared to act as our brain and body building blocks.

Guarding Our Biological Superstructure

Our brain is flesh and blood, and just like other body tissues, it's subjected to wear and tear. The brain's increased energy output creates additional free radicals, which attack this metabolically active organ 24 hours per day, seven days per week.[3] Free radicals are particularly drawn to assaulting fatty tissues, and since our brain is 60 percent fat by weight, it's always on these cellular offenders' radar as a highly appealing target.[4]

Imagine what would happen if we cut an apple in half and allowed it to sit on the counter. In a short time, the sliced portion exposed to the air would turn brown, or oxidize. If we took another apple, cut it in half, but this time squeezed some lemon juice on the exposed surfaces, they would remain fresh looking without much browning or oxidation for a longer period. The antioxidants contained in the lemon juice serve as natural protective preservatives to the apple tissue. Similarly, antioxidants found in plant foods act to guard our brain and other body tissues from dangerous damage.[5]

We can start protecting ourselves by eating foods high in antioxidants—an easy and delicious task most of us have direct control over. Bathing our brain with nutrients that defend it from harmful attacks while promoting exceptional cognitive capacity is essential to reaching our full potential.

A healthy, youthful brain is sustained by antioxidants such as carotenoids found in mangos, apricots, and sweet potatoes; polyphenols found in grapes and berries; selenium from Brazil nuts; vitamin E in nuts and seeds; and vitamin C found in kiwi, red bell pepper, and citrus. In addition, it takes care and fortitude to keep toxins, such as chemically altered foods and known brain poisons, far away from our family's breakfast, lunch, and dinner plates. In the following section, you'll learn which foods to include in your diet for optimal brain health.

Brain-Supporting Foods

Including foods in our diet that contain specific brain-building nutrients is critical to facilitating the best mental function and performance. By actively seeking out and incorporating whole plant foods that specifically contain valuable components, we ensure that our brain is provided with the critical building blocks that enhance its invaluable tasks. Take a look at the following foods and consciously seek to include them in your diet for optimal brain health.

— **Berries:** In the scientific community, these are often referred to as "brain berries" because they contain nutrients that can enhance neural communication within the brain while also helping to repair existing damage.[6] These fruits contain high levels of antioxidants.[7] Anthocyanins, members of the flavonoid group of phytochemicals, have demonstrated the ability to protect against a myriad of human diseases.[8] Anthocyanins are pigments that give fruits, berries, and vegetables their vibrant colors. Think of them as protective mixtures that work to help reduce inflammation and improve immune responses in our brain and body.[9] They show particular promise in cancer research, as trials have indicated their potential to reduce cancer-cell growth while inhibiting tumor formation.[10]

Tasty berries can be easily incorporated into smoothies, slow-cooked oatmeal (not instant), or fruit salads, or be enjoyed by the handful at any time. Frozen berries are good to keep on hand to use during the winter. You can also immerse them in hot (not boiling) water to make tasty tea. During hot weather, making a large pitcher of iced berry tea provides a refreshing, antioxidant-filled drink that can be savored all day. Enjoy blueberries, bilberries, blackberries, raspberries, strawberries, and boysenberries as a delicious, brain-building treat.

— **Fruits:** The antioxidants found in fruits and vegetables have been positively linked to increased cognitive function.[11] Fruits rich in carotenoids such as mangos, apricots, and cantaloupes are tasty and an easy way to invite more brain cellular protection into our day. There are more than 600 different types of carotenoids. Some of the most popularly known include lycopene (found in tomatoes, watermelon, pink grapefruit, papaya, and guava), lutein (found in kiwi and grapes), and beta-carotene (found in apricots, papaya, and mango). Lycopene may help decrease the risk of stroke.[12] The great news about consuming delicious fruits is that most also contain generous amounts of vitamin C, a powerful antioxidant,[13] along with many other vitamins and minerals. Add pomegranate seeds to smoothies and salads, put papayas in fruit salads, and squeeze fresh lemon juice into water and herbal tea. Even small, seemingly insignificant amounts all add up to big antioxidant protection throughout the day.

— **Vegetables:** This category, particularly leafy greens, is abundant in brain-protecting antioxidants such as carotenoids, vitamin C, vitamin E, and selenium. Carotenoid-containing vegetables include yellow and red peppers, carrots, and sweet potatoes (starchy vegetables). Sweet potatoes contain the potent antioxidants, vitamins, and polyphenols that fight inflammation and age-associated degeneration. Lutein, a pigment found in kale, broccoli, and many other fruits and vegetables, has been shown to be a powerful antioxidant and protectant.[14] Including those high in vitamin K from the cruciferous family such as cauliflower and kale decreases oxidative stress inflammation and influences cognitive function.

Eating lots of vegetables and exploring their huge variety is both nutritious and delicious. By centering daily meals around a cornucopia of rainbow-colored veggies, we'll not only enjoy tantalizing flavors, we'll also receive a wide variety of antioxidants and rich plant nutrients.

— **Nuts and seeds:** Along with avocados, these are good sources of vitamin E, which is an important fat-soluble vitamin for normal brain function and the protection of brain cells.[15] Nuts and seeds are also good sources of the fatty acids that are critical for optimal brain function. Incorporating a small handful (one to two ounces or less) of nuts or seeds into our day helps ensure that we get what we need. Enjoy Brazil nuts, walnuts, pecans, almonds, pumpkin seeds, sesame seeds, sunflower seeds, sacha inchi seeds, ground flaxseeds, chia seeds, or others. Be sure to eat nuts raw and unsalted. Chew them well to a creamy consistency before swallowing for better digestion and absorption. Sprinkling a few on salads or tossing a couple into a smoothie adds healthy fats that help with the absorption of nutrients.

— **Choline-rich plant foods:** Choline is an important brain nutrient needed to synthesize the neurotransmitter acetylcholine, which allows the brain and nervous system to function optimally, aiding memory. Good sources include soy foods, quinoa, broccoli, green peas, brussels sprouts, pinto beans, and almonds. Adding quinoa to rice dishes often adds a nuttier, tastier flavor.

— **B vitamin–rich plant foods:** There are numerous B vitamins, and all play an important role in overall health. They're critical for regulating the nervous system, particularly the brain. Vitamin B12 is of special importance because it assists folate in making DNA and RNA, which transmit genetic information to every living cell in our body. B12 also plays a role in the production of the myelin sheath that surrounds nerve fibers. Without enough of this vitamin, nerve transmission suffers and potential nerve damage can result. The best sources of B vitamins are green leafy vegetables, whole grains, legumes (such as beans, peas, and lentils), nuts, and seeds. For proper brain health, I advise supplementation with vitamin B12 to ensure adequate levels.

Quenching the Thirsty Brain

Our brain works around the clock and requires more water than any other part of the body.[16] The brain is about 80 percent water by volume, so even experiencing a slight hydration problem can have negative cognitive consequences due to decreased oxygen delivery. Consistent and prolonged lack of water can cause brain-cell shrinkage and may result in brain injury.

The bloodstream is often referred to as the "river of life" because it carries red blood cells that contain life-sustaining oxygen from the lungs throughout the body and, in particular, to our oxygen-hungry brain. Our brain cannot survive without oxygen even for short periods of time, even when we sleep, without suffering damage and ultimately death.

As we lie down to rest for the night, we cease consuming liquids for a long stretch of time, anywhere from six to eight hours or more. However, the body is still using existing water stores through respiration, sweating, digesting food, and other essential bodily processes. If we don't replenish quality liquids adequately, we risk becoming dehydrated.

A liquid called the cerebral spinal fluid surrounds the brain. This clear secretion originates deep within the brain and provides support, suspending the organ in place as it buoyantly floats within it, acting as a cushion against shock (hitting the head on an object or other potential trauma).

This fluid also transports waste material out and away from our vulnerable brain, decreasing the risk of free-radical harm to this marvel of nature. This is one of the reasons proper hydration is critically important, particularly upon waking in the morning, since ingesting liquids makes oxygen delivery more efficient. Restocking body water levels becomes crucial because it helps thin the blood and ensures rapid oxygen flow to our thirsty cells. This need for liquid should always be met *first*. Hydrating with water, herbal tea, smoothies, juicy fruits, or diluted juices provides the brain and body with the liquids necessary to start the day.

Adding a small amount of pure juice (without artificial ingredients) such as blueberry, cherry, or cranberry to water increases the antioxidants in our diet. In addition, the sweet taste encourages us to drink more. Having undiluted, concentrated juice in the morning may tax the body with too much sugar and slow the absorption of water. Significantly diluted juices help avoid a blood-sugar crash while also preventing us from getting too many calories.

My philosophy regarding fluid consumption is to *maximize every sip* by adding more protective nutrients to the liquid, creating a powerful, enriched elixir. These life enhancers include: fresh green juices (or green powders mixed with clean water), herbs and herbal teas (my clients enjoy Numi brand), spices, and diluted berry juices. Remember to continue to hydrate during the day by taking a chilled smoothie or green powder ready to be mixed (or premixed) with water on the road, to work, and for sipping throughout the day.

Boosting Our Wits

The brain continues to use energy while we sleep (technically, it *never* sleeps). Upon waking, it seeks to restore energy reserves from the nightly fast. The morning meal is called "breakfast" because we've been abstaining from eating during sleep.

People often feel groggy in the morning because they skip breakfast and consequently miss out on fueling the brain. Optimal cognitive functioning should start soon after we awaken and continue throughout the day, but many are ignoring the brain's needs and experience inadequate mental function as a result.

A nourishing morning meal is imperative to rev up the brain and increase energy levels. Fruits, vegetables, smoothies, warm veggie soups (during cold weather), slow-cooked oatmeal (not instant), cooked barley, and other wholesome choices should be the focus early in the day.

The goal is to boost our wits and supply our brain with nutrients. Eating processed foods along with high-fat meals in the morning is particularly insulting to a needy brain seeking quality, nutrient-filled support. Most denatured breakfast fare offers a quick high that's shortly replaced by a deep low, forcing us to seek out snacks to tide us over until lunch.

Stick with whole, unprocessed foods in the morning, and try to make breakfast an important habit. If you find yourself pressed for time, fruit is a great choice. Eating an apple or pear requires only a quick wash (which can be done the night before). Enjoying a quickly prepared bowl of fresh berries with dairy-free cultured coconut milk (my clients enjoy the brand So Delicious) takes moments and provides the brain fuel and protection we need to start the day off right.

Essential Fats for Brain Health

The brain looks for healthy fats to create healthy cell membranes. If we present our brain with unhealthy fats (such as trans fats), it will build structures out of these undesirable fats. This is quite serious as it *directly compromises the integrity of the cell membrane*. It's similar to building our house out of tin cans instead of bricks or cement—not a desirable situation.

Our brain relies on us to supply it with quality, *unprocessed* fats found in whole foods such as fruits, vegetables, nuts, seeds, whole grains, and legumes. These naturally occurring fats are essential to building and repairing cells, both in the brain and throughout the body. If the right nutrients are lacking, critical neurotransmitters will not form and optimal brain functioning will cease. This lack of neurotransmitter support is one of the reasons many children and adults are experiencing overwhelming emotional and behavior problems today.

Our bodies create fatty acids from the foods we consume. One of these essential omega-3 fatty acids is called docosahexaenoic acid (DHA). The highest concentrations of omega-3s is found in our brain.[17] This gives us an important clue about their importance for mental and neurological functioning.

When we consume foods such as ground flaxseeds, walnuts, sacha inchi seeds (grown in the Amazon Rainforest, available from Vega, and one of the best plant sources of omega fatty acids), and green leafy vegetables, our body is able to convert the shorter omega-3 fatty acids these plant foods contain into DHA.

DHA is necessary for reducing inflammation and creating the myelin sheath around our nerves. It also improves vision, the immune system, and memory.[18] Alzheimer's patients have dramatically lower levels of DHA in the neurons of their hippocampus (the brain area responsible for memory). Inadequate amounts can alter dopamine (a neurotransmitter) levels in the brain, leading to problems with attention and learning.[19] Many of my clients with cognitive issues found additional supplementation of DHA from the NuTru brand to be helpful with improving memory and concentration.

Since neurotransmitters require good amino acids, consuming sufficient amounts of beans, peas, and lentils is also important in supporting optimal brain function.

As I explained, essential fats help make up our cells' permeable membrane. This barrier is responsible for keeping undesirable and harmful poisons out of the cell while allowing in good nutrients and cell "helpers." Imagine the membrane as a security officer who guards a cell. If the officer becomes weak, tired, or dysfunctional, bad guys (toxins) may be allowed in to cause destruction, while good guys (nutrients) may be unintentionally kept out. If our security is compromised, the integrity of our cells is affected.

The myelin sheath, the cover that surrounds many nerve cells, increases the speed that information travels along the nerve. The sheath is made up of approximately 70 percent fat and 30 percent protein. Since our brain and spinal cord contain a tremendous number of nerves, if the myelin sheath is damaged, the impulses are no longer transmitted quickly and efficiently, and we start experiencing cognitive decline and neurological problems.

Vitamin B12 is also critical to building the myelin sheath, and helping repair nerve fibers in the brain. High homocysteine (an amino acid) levels may decrease brain function, and B12 helps decrease homocysteine blood levels, aiding cognitive performance.

PS . . . That's Helpful

Phosphatidylserine (PS) is another abundant fat in the brain. It's a fatty acid that helps build brain-cell membranes, making them fluid enough to release the neurotransmitters acetylcholine and dopamine. Unfortunately, PS levels tend to decline with age, an effect worsened by deficiencies in other fatty acids, folic acid, and vitamin B12.

PS supplementation, under the advice of a qualified health professional, may help brain-cell membranes, stimulate nerve cell growth, lower stress hormones, and assist in generating new connections between cells, helping to prevent cognitive decline.[20] PS has also been shown to influence tissue response to inflammation and act as an effective antioxidant.

As PS is reduced, the ability to learn, remember, and stay mentally alert is decreased. This fatty acid has shown promise in treating Alzheimer's disease and dementia.[21] PS efficiency is enhanced in the presence of DHA,[22] making the pair, along with other cofactors, synergistic partners in brain health. It's crucially important when buying PS to make sure that it's derived from soy lecithin and not cow brains (a huge concern because of mad cow disease). My clients have benefited greatly from the PS supplement P-Tidyl-Weil from NuTru. Other sources of PS include white beans and soy beans.

Fabricated Fats

Certain fats are particularly detrimental to brain health and should be avoided. Trans fats, the "twisted sisters" of our body's healthy fats, make the top of the undesirables list. When hydrogen is added to oil, the mixture turns from a liquid to a solid. This artificial concoction is a blessing to food manufacturers, who profit from the cheap technique that increases the texture of foods as well as prolonging their shelf life. Unfortunately for the consumer, the newly made hydrogenated product increases the production of low-density lipoprotein (LDL), the bad cholesterol that increases our risk of coronary heart disease.[23]

It's currently mandated that foods containing trans fat be labeled in the U.S. However, if a product serving contains 0.5 grams or less of this ingredient, it can be legally labeled as *zero*.[24] This means that if a package of chips contains four servings and has one and a half grams of trans fat, it can be labeled as zero since it's less than 0.5 grams *per serving*. Do we know anyone who's ever stopped at eating one serving of chips? Most people crunch down half the package or more. This makes the trans fat consumption greater than the amount considered safe—namely, none.

The FDA estimates that Americans eat close to six grams of trans fat *per day*. The National Academy of Sciences (NAS) has concluded that there is *no safe level* of this substance. Furthermore, trans fat has been linked to Alzheimer's disease, cancer, diabetes, obesity, liver dysfunction, infertility, cardiovascular risks, and depression. As much as 40 percent of the foods on grocery-store shelves contain trans fats, making avoiding these undesirable fats challenging but achievable with a bit of forethought, knowledge, and persistence.

The key is to focus on eating more fresh, wholesome fruits and vegetables and pass on products containing processed fat, such as margarine; shortening; donuts; pies; most instant popcorn; and many breakfast cereals, granola bars, cookies, and crackers. *Run* from products that contain these words in their ingredient list: *partially hydrogenated, hydrogenated,* and any words that are difficult to pronounce, you need a pharmaceutical dictionary to define, or require an advance degree in chemistry to recognize.

Nutritional Strategies for Aggression

It seems as if we're living in an increasingly angry world. Aggression has now become a way of life for many children and adults for several important reasons: First, we're continually bombarded with senseless and glorified violence in the media, including television, movies, books, and video games. Simply witnessing aggressive behavior sparks similar tendencies in observers.[25] Now imagine taking young, vulnerable children and immersing them in violent video games disguised as innocent play, every day for hours. Second, add severe deficiencies in nutrients essential for brain function (compliments of the Standard American Diet), and we have a formula for mental, emotional, physiological, and ultimately, social disaster.

Becoming mindful of providing the brain with essential fatty acids such as DHA and EPA (eicosapentaenoic acid), along with synergistic nutrients such as B12 and others, helps the brain regain its equilibrium and health. Both DHA and EPA have been shown to benefit attention deficit disorder and aggression.[26] These should be considered and explored for addressing anger and hostility. Essential fatty acids also generate neuro-protective effects, offering critical defense support to cell membranes.

Jeff's Story

Jeff's parents brought him to my office several years ago because he was suffering from severe attention deficit disorder, hyperactivity, extreme aggression, and frightening violence. Although he was only 18 years old, Jeff had already been to nine psychologists and six psychiatrists. Trying every prescribed brain medication under the sun without finding any relief, Jeff was put on experimental medications. When these failed to work, he was referred to me as a last hope. Working in conjunction with his doctor, I suggested that Jeff try DHA, PS, and vitamin B12 supplementation. I also changed his diet by filling it with high-nutrient, whole plant matter. DHA has been shown to be helpful in cases of aggression and ADD,[27] and B12 is essential for proper brain function. Other B vitamins were also included for brain support. Jeff also stopped listening to antagonistic music and playing violent video games.

In a short time, people started coming up to Jeff's parents asking about the miracle that healed their son. He became calm and relaxed, and continued getting better month after month. No longer controlled by aggression, Jeff was now feeling peaceful, content, and serene. Since he avoided music with violent lyrics and gruesome video games, his aggression exposure was limited, which helped him significantly. Today, Jeff is doing tremendously well and continues to take his supplements. He comments on feeling the difference if he forgets his DHA, PS, and B12 and feels best when sticking with his protocol.

Spice Is Wise for the Brain

One of the most important strategies I encourage my clients to implement is found in everyone's kitchen: spices. With little more than a shake or two of the wrist, we can incorporate super-concentrated nutrients while making unique taste enhancements to any dish. Throughout history, spices were used predominantly to prevent bacterial and fungal growth in foods since refrigeration did not exist. Spices essentially perform the same antioxidant miracles on the brain and body. Adding delightful aromas and color that enhance our interest, spices and herbs can be used fresh or dried, making them versatile in cooking. They're of particular importance due to their potency and the concentration of compounds essential for brain care and preservation. Ounce for ounce, spices and herbs contain the greatest quantity of antioxidant protection.[28]

Incorporating specific spices into daily meals makes eating more enjoyable and adds concentrated nutrients to our body and brain. My favorite "brain spices" for clients are cinnamon, rosemary, turmeric, mint, ginger, and basil. There are, of course, many others, but I find that my chosen top six are the most readily available, commonly recognized, versatile, and universally appealing. I urge everyone to explore the spices in their cupboards and look up the benefits in books and online. The more merit we find in ingesting the spices we love, the greater our chances of adding them to our meals consistently.

— **Cinnamon:** Obtained from the bark of a tree, cinnamon has been known to help stabilize blood-glucose levels, improve triglycerides, and lower cholesterol. It also has an anti-inflammatory effect in the brain and body,[29] and is antiviral and antifungal. This spice has been highly effective in helping my clients keep blood-sugar levels steady throughout the day. High blood-sugar levels can assault and damage the arteries, leading to cognitive decline. Many of my clients have enjoyed foods more by adding this remarkable spice to their diet. A great technique is mixing one-quarter to one-half teaspoon of cinnamon into various dishes. It can be easily sprinkled into herbal tea, fruit, and smoothies. Smelling cinnamon essential oil has been shown to promote greater attention span and memory. Choose Ceylon cinnamon over cassia or Chinese varieties. If you're taking medication, be sure to check with a qualified professional before trying cinnamon since it can change the dosage necessary to maintain blood-glucose levels.

— **Rosemary:** This flavorful spice helps with cognitive enhancement.[30] It's an anti-inflammatory, which is important in preventing dementia. Extremely versatile, rosemary can be used in food dishes or sipped as a tea. You can also toss a pinch of fresh rosemary into smoothies for a unique taste treat. Smelling the essential oil of rosemary throughout the workday has provided many of my clients with the stimulation needed to accomplish intellectually tedious tasks and avoid mental exhaustion. Rosemary complements potato dishes and most tomato-based sauces.

— **Turmeric:** Curry lovers will be thrilled to hear that turmeric is a prominent spice in most curry mixtures (along with mustard), accounting for their vibrant, signature yellow color. Turmeric is a powerful brain-cell protectant and an overall strong antioxidant and anti-inflammatory agent. That's vitally important for brain neurons. Scientists have been studying residents in rural India to determine the reasons for their low incidence of Alzheimer's disease. It's believed that the rhizomes (root stalks) of the turmeric plant contain powerful compounds that help brain function, along with curcumin.[31] Not to be confused with the spice cumin, this is just one of the nine curcuminoids contained in turmeric, all of which are highly protective to the body, particularly the brain. Turmeric contains anti-amyloid properties. Beta-amyloid protein is a sticky substance that can accumulate in the brain and prevent neurons from communicating with each other; too much of it is believed to play a role in causing Alzheimer's symptoms. Curcumin seems to reduce the damaging effect of protein plaque in Alzheimer's patients, while reliving oxidative stress caused by free radicals.[32] Turmeric is delicious with potatoes, lentils, rice, soups, and most vegetables. You can enhance the absorption of curcumin by adding black pepper to curry dishes.

— **Mint:** This refreshing herb has long been used for stomach upset. Highly revered for its antibacterial and antifungal properties,[33] mint is important for brain health because it assists the body in scavenging for dangerous free radicals.[34] Its refreshing taste can sweeten our breath and add zesty flavor to salads and vegetables. Mint tea is also popular for digestive discomfort, flatulence, and overall digestive health. Adding finely chopped mint leaves to guacamole is a surprisingly delicious treat.

— **Ginger:** A welcome spice for those with nausea and stomach issues, ginger root can be used extensively in food dishes, as a tea, and in aromatherapy formulations. It contains anti-inflammatory compounds that are important to brain and body function.[35] It also lessens the depletion of glutathione, one of the body's most important internally produced antioxidants. Ginger can be enjoyed grated in most dishes and soups for a spicy, rich flavor, and ginger tea is popular for soothing the nerves and assisting digestion; a dash of ginger in smoothies adds flavorful zest. The dried, ground spice is fine when fresh isn't available.

— **Basil:** This herb has been shown to provide protection against bacterial growth, act as an anti-inflammatory,[36] and decrease free-radical damage. Important for brain health, fresh basil is delicious in pesto, salads, and vegetable dishes. A few fresh leaves dropped in a cool pitcher of water add a delightfully fresh flavor. Smelling a sprig of basil or the essential oil has been helpful in decreasing headaches due to tension and tight muscles since basil promotes muscle relaxation.[37]

Focusing on brain-building whole foods and spices helps provide the nutritional support necessary for optimal cognitive functioning. In the following chapter, you'll learn the importance of brain exercises that promote greater mental fitness.

CHAPTER 5

FLEXING MENTAL MUSCLES

Our brain, similar to our muscles, requires oxygen, nutrients, and stimulation for optimal functioning. Just as our physical performance increases with different and challenging fitness routines, the brain also benefits from mental "cross-training" to expand its problem-solving skills, memory, and creativity. The mind can become complacent after a while, doing the same activities day in and day out. Not presenting unique stimuli can cause it to wither, much like a flower going without water for long durations. The more we exercise the brain in unique and unusual ways, the more we flourish by enjoying its increased capabilities.

More than 20 years ago, I was inspired to create some of the first comprehensive "brain building" classes in the country. My focus was threefold: To educate everyone about nutrition's role in brain health, to encourage physical movement, and to challenge the mind with unusual and stimulating exercises. I soon became a regular speaker at retirement homes, senior centers, and adult day-care facilities around the country. The audiences typically walked into the class somewhat lethargic, but they quickly perked up when they heard the fast-paced music I had playing and smelled the aromatherapy scents I sprayed in the air. I would instruct as often as three times per week at individual senior centers or retirement homes. Teaching these classes over the decades provided me with a unique opportunity to witness people's transformations and progress. It allowed me to gain many valuable insights into the workings of the brain and, in particular, memory. Not surprisingly, these sessions became extremely popular and highly requested, and soon required more and more time and dedication.

Our elderly population, especially those in care facilities, spends a great deal of time being sedentary and relatively little time engaged in activities that promote greater cognitive function. When I challenged seniors with games and activities, improved their physical fitness, and fine-tuned their diet, their health increased, along with their mental faculties—sometimes significantly. They began to get excited about learning. A few of the dietary additions I recommended included: sprinkling ground flaxseeds on top of their oatmeal to help reduce inflammation and improve brain function, eating blueberries to help enhance neuronal communication and repair damage that may have occurred in the brain, and adding one-quarter to one-half teaspoon of cinnamon to help reduce blood-sugar levels. Hydration was also a priority, along with keeping the diet lower in fat.

After interviewing actively fit and thriving seniors from all over the country, I found some key modalities in their life: First, none had grown up with the technology we have today. In many ways, this was a blessing. Since they didn't posses computers, their brains had to do the computing. Universally, I found that seniors were exceptional with numbers because they didn't have calculators at a young age. Second, without the constant distraction of television, they exchanged stories, played games (such as cards, chess, checkers, *Monopoly, Scrabble,* Ping-Pong, and bowling), and reminisced about their favorite memories for entertainment. This stimulated the brain and paved the way for good cognitive function into their later years.

Even though our technology has progressed through time, it does not mean that our diet has. Many of our eating habits have taken a drastic step backward. Seniors of yesterday were spared from many of the food and environmental contaminants I talked about earlier. Additionally, almost all the seniors I spoke with described a physically active lifestyle in their childhood. Many walked miles to get to school and back home, rain or shine. Some even carried younger siblings on their back during their long foot commutes.

I encouraged seniors to get back into walking, especially before having breakfast, to stimulate their circulation. Movement increases blood flow to the brain and throughout the body, activating endorphins and helping us with motivation. I stressed the importance of drinking diluted juices upon waking to help hydrate the body after sleeping.

It's fun and enjoyable to engage the mind and senses with music, aromatherapy, and games. I frequently distributed "homework," which we went over at the next class, and some people became so inspired they stayed up during the evening trying to figure out puzzles, riddles, and mathematical problems. That was exactly my goal: to have them use the brain all the time. I still keep the heartfelt letters and testimonials I received from seniors whose lives had dramatically improved because of these classes.

In the following sections, you'll gain tools and strategies to challenge, strengthen, and expand your mind. As you become more diligent in providing your brain with its own required form of calisthenics, you'll benefit from its increased mental abilities.

Brain Cross-Training

If I asked you to solve a crossword puzzle today, your brain would be stretched to find the answers. However, if I gave you the same puzzle tomorrow and the next day, the strain of finding solutions would be less and less taxing because your brain would be used to the questions and know most of the answers from repetition and practice. If you continued to lift light weights when you worked your arm muscles, you'd eventually stop seeing progress. Similarly, challenging your brain by solving problems, thinking "outside the box," and tackling brain puzzles, helps it "flex" and stay cognitively fit.

Try the following suggestions to improve mental abilities and challenge the brain:

- Use your non-dominant hand, leg, or appendage every day in a *safe* way. Write your name, push a button, and eat with the opposite hand (but don't try to drive a car or pick up hot liquids with the non-dominant hand).

- Read materials that may be more difficult and mentally demanding than your usual selections. If you read the sports section frequently, change it up and try the cooking feature first. If business news gets ignored, stimulate your brain by reading it anyway.

- Expanding your vocabulary is one of the best ways to challenge the brain. Try to learn a few new words every day, as well as their meanings, and use them daily in conversations.

- Challenge the brain with puzzles and games. Invest time in board games, online or printed puzzles, or television trivia shows. When watching a trivia show, try to figure out the answers before the contestants.

- Attempt to learn a foreign language. Even looking up a few new words and using them throughout the day is beneficial.

- Use scents to engage the brain. Memories from decades prior can be evoked simply by recognizing certain smells. I'll talk more about the importance of smell in the coming sections.

- Make up fun exercises such as reciting the months of the year in alphabetical order; counting by twos (2, 4, 6, 8) and then counting backward (8, 6, 4, 2); and later changing the factor number to five (5, 10, 15), and then counting down backwards with the same factor number (15, 10, 5).

- Keep a pen and paper handy while watching television. When the commercials begin, try to make a list from memory of the last scenes you viewed before the commercial. Jot down details such as colors of furnishing; what the actors were wearing; and any flowers, paintings, and rugs in the scene.

- An hour before going to bed, write down a list of all the significant happenings of the day: 9 A.M.: read a great article on brain health, 10 A.M.: worked on project, 11 A.M.: conference call, 12 P.M.: ate a nutritious vegetable salad, and so on.

- Challenge the brain by seeking to incorporate one new fruit or vegetable into the day. If you haven't eaten a grapefruit in years, buy one today. Explore new and unusual produce such as star fruit or lychee—look at the produce section of the store with new eyes.

MIND for Brain Health

I came up with an easy acronym you can use to remember how to incorporate good brain health habits into your daily life: MIND.

— **Movement:** A healthy brain requires good circulation; it must have oxygen, and a stronger heart can pump more oxygenated blood throughout the body. The arteries should be clear and unclogged, with good diameters, allowing for sufficient blood flow. Moving the body frequently during the day, even for short periods of time, helps to keep oxygen supplied to the brain. If you're feeling stuck on a mental problem while sitting at work, simply standing up and walking around for a few minutes should get the circulation moving and will help you think better. Many people find that taking a short stroll and stretching helps the brain find new solutions to challenges.

— **Imagination:** Provide the brain with interesting ideas, thoughts, and intellectual data to stimulate increased cognitive function. Creatively engage your mind in solving various problems and seek solutions with new and imaginative possibilities. Continue this stimulation daily with unique, unusual, and challenging games, concepts, and learning. Expand your imagination by thinking "outside the box."

— **Nutrition:** Excellent nutrition, along with proper hydration, is crucial for brain nourishment and protection. When the diet is high in fat, it causes slow, sludgy movement of oxygen. Focus on including fresh, whole plant foods brimming with vitamins, minerals, antioxidants, and fiber. Remember to consume brain-building foods and spices daily.

— **Delight:** Seek to be delighted and find enjoyment in the day. Happiness and laughter reduce blood pressure and releases endorphins, bathing our brain in feel-good chemicals. Find ways to delight the people around you with kind gestures and words. Being joyous is vital because the brain runs best on happiness. Strive to delight the mind with fun, compassion, and love.

Groovy Habits

Like the chisel a wood carver uses to etch grooves into a piece of wood, our daily habits become the engraving instruments that shape the channels of our mind. When we repeatedly practice the same actions and thoughts, they influence our brain patterns over time. These mental pathways can carry us toward either lackluster mediocrity or joyous vibrancy.

Since our habits seem involuntary, we rarely stop to think about the pivotal role they play. If you take the same route to work every day, after arriving at the office you sometimes can't remember how you got there because you were operating on autopilot. This is one example of how our daily routines become fixed in the brain. The more we train and drill a skill, the more automatic it becomes until we eventually stop thinking about it consciously.

We're biologically prone to follow our most practiced regimens because if we had to make a conscious choice about everything we did during the day, we'd soon become overwhelmed. Activities and even thoughts that require the least amount of effort draw us in because they're undemanding and simple. Fast-food franchises readily take advantage of our tendencies to gravitate toward ease and convenience. Unfortunately, continuing to engage in negative behaviors may pave the way to decreased energy, if they're health depleting.

It takes physical, mental, and emotional energy to overcome poor habits and kick-start a positive routine, but it *can be accomplished* with persistence, patience, and self-love. If we want to stop eating cookies at home, we can donate the boxes in our cupboards and stop buying them. Eating a cookie would then require a trip to the store. This may involve getting dressed, driving, parking, and standing in line. The more energy it takes to obtain undesirable food, the less likely we are to eat it. That's why preparing healthy snacks in advance is so effective. Forward planning dramatically limits our chances of giving in to poor patterns.

Eating a high-calorie, processed-sugar dessert after dinner is a deeply ingrained habit for many of my new clients who want to shed excess fat. One of the methods I use to alter this pattern is simply inviting them to eat three servings of fruit every day. I ask that the first serving be consumed in the morning and the last two be eaten right after dinner. This breaks their automatic routine and allows them to feel satisfied from the sweet, delicious, whole fruit. Their confidence is increased because the goal of refraining from fatty, processed desserts is easily accomplished.

The key to permanent positive change is to create habits that automatically reward us without too much effort. We can stock the refrigerator with sliced fruits and vegetables, making it easier for us to munch on them when we want to snack. I always encourage my clients to make a habit of preparing foods on Sunday for the coming week. Once we've washed and chopped vegetables, cooked grains, and sealed all of it in containers, we have the ready-made ingredients available to quickly put together healthy meals during the busy workweek without much time or energy.

Changing Stuck Patterns

Some of my new clients seek out my assistance specifically because they're stuck in negative habits that are detrimental to their lives. One was a middle-aged man who fell into the routine of going to a bar for alcoholic drinks after work. It began to damage his health, finances, and family life. He desperately wanted to stop, but found that he couldn't because this habit was deeply ingrained in his mind. Because *patterns can be interrupted and changed,* I asked him to stop bringing his cash and credit cards to work and instead to leave them at home. He could still go to the bar if he wanted, but he would have to go home first to pick up his money. This is one of the strategies I implemented as a road-block to help stop his addiction. He agreed to try this approach.

When it was time to leave work at the end of the day, he felt the usual urge (ingrained mental habit) to visit the bar, but couldn't because he didn't have a way to pay for his alcohol. Picking up his money required driving to his house. This meant that if he wanted to go to his favorite bar, he would have to spend more time driving and sitting in traffic. The extra energy this required was like putting a stick inside a wheel; it interrupted his ingrained negative pattern and made it more difficult to accomplish. As he continued to invite the new habit into his daily routine, the old pattern began to dissipate and fade until he no longer felt the urge to go to the bar, even if he had cash in his wallet. Altering the negative pattern had a liberating affect on his self-esteem.

I received an e-mail from him a month later telling me that he had been sober for four weeks. As another month passed, I received another e-mail saying that he was sober going on two months. Finally, a year later, I received an invitation to his one-year celebration of sobriety. He had not set foot inside a bar for a full year. This, along with other pattern interrupters I added into his life, did the job.

Managing Self-Talk

One of the most challenging mental habits is the confidence-splitting and heart-piercing noise of ceaseless negative self-talk. When you put yourself down in a demeaning fashion countless times during the day, this pattern begins to play itself out in your thoughts and, eventually, your actions. This common routine is similar to hearing a jammed CD repeat a recording over and over.

Continually calling yourself degrading names and criticizing every decision takes a damaging toll on your well-being. One method of breaking this gloomy pattern is countering each negative word with three positive ones. If you just called yourself clumsy, immediately say: "I'm coordinated, I'm balanced, and I'm harmonious." This interrupts the harmful self-defeating messages you hear from yourself, replacing them with inspiring and uplifting words that raise your confidence and self-esteem.

If you find yourself stuck in the energy-depleting habit of sitting too much while watching television, you can begin to use the commercial time to get up and do a few physical movements or train your brain with challenging mental exercises. Placing a movable piece of fitness equipment, such as a medicine ball, next to the couch will help serve as a reminder to move more. Keeping a mind-stimulating puzzle or a mentally challenging book next to your chair will similarly encourage you to work your brain muscles during commercials.

While you may be temporarily stuck in some negative habits, you always have the power to change them for the better. Instead of being a victim of past patterns and allowing them to control your life, you can begin to use them as powerful stepping-stones to joyful satisfaction and personal fulfillment. Initiate positive habits with the suggestions in this book, and use mental creativity to create additional healthy routines.

Escaping Boxed Thinking

How much of our day is compartmentalized into physical and mental "boxes"? We sleep in a bed shaped like a box and inhabit a room built like a box, which is inside the bigger container of our home. Our cars are mechanical cartons that transport us to our square cubicles at work, in the larger box of a building. Many people eat processed foods from boxes, which contain items shaped like squares, and then watch programs on box-shaped screens. Life begins to resemble a Russian nesting doll that shuts in our unlimited potential in countless layers of enclosures and dividers.

We've all heard the expression, "Think outside the box," which encourages us to think unconventionally. Yet how often do we eat the same dinner, watch the same show, root for the same team, talk with the same people, read the same newspaper, and follow the same exercise routine day in and day out? Like a clothes dryer that spins our laundry around and around, today looks and feels much like yesterday and the day before.

If we're "boxed in" to our mental patterns, which frequently dictate our routines, we may continue to experience the same monotonous agenda tomorrow, the next day, and for the following months and years. When our mind stops using its abundant *creative ability* to think of unique solutions and ways of doing things, we may continue to engage in the same robotic behaviors for decades. We can do better than that.

Expanding our thinking helps remove the mental limits placed upon us by habits and patterns. We then gain a greater ability to see the bigger picture of our life. Thinking outside the box may be as simple as changing one word in a sentence. For example, some new clients recoil automatically when I ask them to exercise. They associate the word *exercise* with pain, boredom, and frustration. When I substitute the word *movement* and invite them to simply move their body more during the day, they're able to accomplish it with greater ease. Similarly, when certain clients couldn't fathom taking a "wimpy salad" to work with them for lunch because they were used to hearty sandwiches, I simply suggested they place many vegetables between large pieces of chard, lettuce leaves, or brown-rice tortillas and wrap it all together. Then they were able to eat hearty "salad sandwiches" without any trouble. People who don't like to eat vegetables can generally enjoy them in smoothies, and a salad can become a green smoothie if we start expanding our thinking with imagination and creativity. The result is virtually the same—eating more veggies—but the method used to accomplish the goal is inspired by unconventional thinking.

Perhaps one of the best examples of someone who personified revolutionary thinking is Bruce Lee. A renowned martial artist and a revered philosopher, he looked at martial arts, physical fitness, and life in ways that others dared not because of traditional cultural restraints. When machines didn't exist to help hone his physical skills, he used his creativity and imagination to invent equipment that could increase his strength, speed, and reflexes. When others sought to limit his teachings, he continued to push forward with his vision to make martial arts available to everyone, regardless of outside pressures. If Bruce Lee had bowed to society's dictates or simply given up trying to think in an unorthodox way, we wouldn't enjoy the legacy and principles he left behind.

Consider the following tips as inspiration to expand your thinking.

Tips to Think Outside the Box

- Look for a new route to get to work or home.
- Open your mind to communicating and building friendships with people of all ages without judgment.
- Come up with new ways to accomplish things. Break the rules of mental thought and explore creative solutions to everyday challenges.
- Become curious about various topics. If math was not an interest for you in the past, look for books about numbers that could be interesting and see if you can

get into learning some of the information. You may surprise yourself and enjoy a subject you thought you disliked only because you misunderstood it or because it wasn't explained well in the past.

- Just because an idea sounds silly, it doesn't mean that it's not useful. Look to unusual and "foolish" ideas as the stepping-stones to fresh new solutions.

- Embrace daydreaming, which is a right-brain, mind-expanding, creativity-liberating activity.

- Think in groundbreaking and pioneering ways. Bring up different viewpoints and introduce creative solutions to problems.

- Invest in free time, which is all too frequently missing in life. This is when we can be spontaneous and creative and try different activities.

- Encourage kids to spend time with seniors and share stories, ideas, and life experiences. Both generations can benefit greatly from learning from each other.

By exploring these mind-expanding ideas, your creativity will flourish and you'll begin to enjoy greater cognitive function. Remember to flex your mental muscles often. Challenge your brain daily and appreciate its increased capabilities. In the next chapter, I'll share some of my favorite brain-enhancing modalities, and you'll learn how to incorporate them into your life easily and joyfully.

CHAPTER 6

BRAIN-ENHANCING MODALITIES

You've learned the importance of nourishing the brain with nutritious foods and the significant effect of challenging your mind with brain-building exercises and unconventional thinking. In this chapter, I'll focus on showing you how several modalities can greatly enhance your cognitive function in ways that are easily doable and enjoyable. You'll notice that, along with cognitive performance, your moods will also see improvements and you'll experience increased emotional balance.

That's Music to My Brain

Our brain is divided into two recognizable hemispheres, the right and the left. These distinct areas communicate with each other through bands consisting of millions of nerve fibers. Each hemisphere is thought to be dominant in certain abilities. The left side of the brain controls muscles on the right side of the body and governs certain traits such as language, solving math problems, and logic. The right side of the brain specializes in recognizing faces, visualizing, daydreaming, and music. We can think of the left side of the brain as the math genius who budgets our finances to the penny and the right side as the creative, imaginative artist who draws inspired flowers and innovative shapes on the same checkbook.

We function well when we use both hemispheres, much like using both sides of our body. Unfortunately, today's left-brain-focused society structures our existence to revolve around rigid thinking at the expense of consistently engaging our visionary right brain. This is similar to tying our right hand behind our back and using only the left; the result is imbalance and the impairment of our full potential.

Our children are being pulled into left-brain thinking earlier and earlier in life. Parents want their children to get a head start on our rapidly changing world, so the strict academia often begins while kids are still in diapers. The indoctrination into fact-based learning—which limits imagination, artistry, and innovation—continues to dominate our existence from cradle to grave.

Children now receive less and less music instruction in schools because funding these programs is often last on the list of priorities. This is quite sad because children are missing out on one of the most profoundly effective methods of stimulating the right brain (not to mention the enjoyment music brings). Most important, music is a form of self-expression. It allows us to convey who we are and what we feel in an individual manner.

The right brain seeks to make invaluable contributions even when it's ignored and disused. It's frequently responsible for committing school-day offenses such as daydreaming and doodling on paper. After years of dominant left-brain thinking, the right brain begins to perform like an atrophied limb that has been tightly constricted in a cast. Regaining full function takes time, practice, and self-love.

Beginning to wake up our right brain starts with a powerful method of exercising and strengthening it to function better: music. Our nervous system makes associations between complex sounds and their meaning—it's like mental gymnastics. Simply listening to music can be beneficial because it stimulates specific regions of the brain responsible for memory, language, and motor control.

Music can also help lower our heart rate and decrease anxiety. Almost every movie we watch has a score that, often unnoticed, plays in the background to evoke certain emotions and magnify the desired effects of the images. Watching a scary movie with the sound muted suddenly makes us less frightened, and lowering the volume during commercials dampens their impact.

Music can be used as a powerful therapy for communication and self-expression for those who feel withdrawn. It can become the medium that releases emotions that are difficult to convey in words.

Learning to play an instrument affects memory, attention, language, and fine motor communication. Musical training tones the brain for listening effectively.[1] Actively working with sounds enhances neuroplasticity, the ability of the brain to adapt to change.[2] It's fun to play, and people around us love to hear familiar and new melodies. There are numerous ways to get started. For example, community colleges and local park districts often offer a variety of classes. If you have an instrument at home that's gathering dust from disuse, you can pick it up and practice playing for several minutes every day to help engage the brain.

Exciting research also indicates that music affects levels of cortisone, testosterone, and estrogen, improving the mood states of people with psychiatric disorders, Parkinson's, and Alzheimer's disease.[3] Listening to and practicing playing music helps our body increase its well-being and should be considered a powerful brain-enhancing modality.

Musical Mantras

Children often learn the alphabet as a song because *music helps the brain retain facts*. This can have positive or negative effects. When we want to memorize something complex, music is particularly effective because the rhythms, rhymes, and attractive melodies spur our mental engagement. But if we continually listen to music with angry or violent lyrics, the result may be detrimental.

How many times do we catch ourselves with the same tune in our head during the day? Lyrics, when listened to countless times, often become "subconscious mantras." If we usually listen to music that spews hate and destruction, it will have an impact on our thoughts. Many kids become influenced by music that encourages brutality and hate. This should be avoided, even if it's promoted as popular and fun.

My experience in working with violent teenagers has shown that eliminating music with abusive and cruel lyrics dramatically decreased these kids' inclinations toward aggressive behavior. Once they switched to calming, soothing options, such as classical music, they became more peaceful and serene. When they began to spend time with friends who listened to vicious lyrics, they began to exhibit violent behavior again.

Becoming conscious of what we play or hear is important because of the effect on our moods, thoughts, and eventually, behaviors. Music has a powerful influence on the brain and is not to be taken lightly. It's a wonderful catalyst for healing and learning and should be explored and enjoyed for its unlimited potential.

The Gems Under Our Nose

Smell is one of the first things we notice when entering a new place. Every breath we take monitors our surroundings for possible danger or potential pleasure. Our noses are so sensitive that they can recognize and process more than ten thousand different scents.

Odors are volatile molecules that float through the air. As we inhale, they rush into our nostrils and cause our brain to perceive, in milliseconds, what information needs to be sent to our bloodstream and neocortex. Being the only sense with receptor nerve endings in direct contact with the outside world, smell provides a direct channel to our brain.[4]

Scent is a powerful means of communication with our environment and each other. It alerts us to toxic chemicals, spoiled food, fresh flowers, and the presence of loved ones. The most direct and profound impression we have of others is their aroma. We sometimes say, "That just doesn't smell right to me," when expressing uneasiness about a situation because we instinctually recognize that smell is associated with feelings.

Our memories and moods are deeply and profoundly affected by odors. They stimulate long-term recall as no other sense can and give us direct access to our emotions because smells *don't require language.*

Odors immediately affect us because they pass the blood-brain barrier (the membrane that sheathes and protects the brain). Large molecules cannot pass this protective blockade, but oxygen and some nutrients can. Different odors stimulate different brain centers to release neurochemicals that affect us in a number of ways.

One of the first things I noticed while working in geriatrics was the impaired sense of smell in our senior population. Because our sense of taste is greatly affected by smell, when the nasal passages are clogged because of a cold, an allergy, or the flu, or are damaged by smoking and other environmental pollutants, appetite is frequently lost because we can't detect odors well. Many seniors lose their appetite because of impared smell, and this can lead to a dangerous situation. Fewer nutrients are offered to the body, making seniors more vulnerable to nutritional deficiencies. Also, the air quality in senior-care facilities (and in many indoor evironments in general) tends to be very poor, making essential-oil use indoors particularly important.

Throughout the years of lecturing in senior-care facilities, I often arrived early and sprayed a mixture of water, rosemary essential oil, and peppermint essential oil around the center and corners of the room. As the seniors entered the space, there was a notable shift for the better in their energy level, and they frequently commented on how wonderful the room smelled.

In the following sections, I'll share how my clients' moods and cognitive ability were helped through the years with the use of essential oils. You'll learn just how easy it is to invite joyful smells into the day and benefit from them.

Smells Good to My Brain

People have used essential oils for thousands of years. Most are derived from the distillation of the leaves, stems, flowers, bark, and roots of plants. The oils are widely utilized today in topical lotions, bath formulas, shampoos, deodorants, toothpastes, aromatherapy products, and a variety of herbal remedies. It's fascinating that the majority of body products on the market mimic the scents of flowers, fruits, vegetables, or herbs. I have yet to encounter lotions that smell like cows, chickens, or pigs. It seems that not only are we attracted to eating fruits, vegetables, greens, and herbs, but we also want to smell more like them.

Each essential oil promotes different feelings and enhances certain mental and physical states. Grapefruit and lemon oils are good for inhaling in the morning, when we wish to be energized and ready to start the day. Cinnamon and peppermint odors have been found to keep drivers more alert while curbing fatigue and frustration behind the wheel.[5]

This is a technique my clients have found to be very effective for recovering from addictions: Relax completely, focus on peaceful and calming thoughts and feelings, and smell an essential oil such as lavender during this serene state. This anchors the essential oil being inhaled to the positive state of mind and helps ensure that the future use of the oil is effective. When clients feel that itch or craving for an addictive substance, they simply pull out their bottle of lavender essential oil and smell it. This takes them back to that calm and peaceful state, breaking the spell of the addictive yearning.

I also encourage my clients to save the peels of citrus such as oranges, tangerines, lemons, or limes (after eating the fruit), and place the peels in small plastic bags. The baggies can be brought to work or used at home or inside the car when a quick pick-me-up is needed. Simply opening the bag, squeezing the peel with your fingers (away from the eyes), and inhaling provides a mental boost with lemon and lime peels, and brings about relaxation with orange and tangerine peels. Everyone benefits from this practice tremendously because it challenges the brain with delightful scents, which helps improve cognitive function.

While my discussion here focuses primarily on the use of essential oils for inhalation, some can also be used for direct skin application (when diluted with a carrier oil) or occasionally for ingestion, under a trained professional's care.

My hope is to inspire everyone to explore the uses of essential oils and learn more about their properties. There are numerous books, websites, and dedicated practitioners who can share valuable information. The Now brand carries organic essential oils that many of my clients enjoy, and other sources can be found in health-food stores and online.

Keep the following tips in mind if you're new to working with essential oils.

Essential Oil Tips

- Be sure to purchase the highest-quality, food-grade oils without artificial ingredients or additives.

- If you're considering trying essential oils externally on the skin, check for allergic reactions first by trying a tiny amount on a small patch of skin and noting any side effects. Stop using immidiately if there are any negative effects. Use a carrier oil or lotion for dilution. When diluting with oil, six drops of essential oil per fluid ounce of carrier oil will yield a one percent solution which is generally regarded as safe for children over three years old.

- Many oils, particularly in the citrus family, are highly phototoxic. This means they contain elements that absorb sunlight intensely, increasing the sun's effect on the skin, which may cause permanent skin disoloration. These oils should not be applied for 48 hours prior to being exposed to sunlight. A partial list of common phototoxic oils includes bergamot, cassia, cumin, ginger, lemon, lime, orange, tangerine, grapefruit, mandarin, and verbena.

- Think, *Less is more,* when it comes to essential oils because they're extremely concentrated. A small drop goes a long way. An easy rule of thumb for diluting the oils with water to spray around a room is to add six drops of essential oil for each fluid ounce of water.

- Change oils every few weeks because the body begins to acclimate to them over time, losing some of the positive effects.

- Never allow essential oils to touch the eyes or mucous membranes.

- Keep oils away from children and out of direct sunlight.

- Be careful if using oils around pets as some may be harmful to their health.

- Consult a professional expert when trying essential oils, especially on the skin or if you're considering using them internally.

Enjoying Essential Oils

If I had to choose the most versatile and useful essential oils for the average home and medicine cabinet, the following ten would be my favorites. Keep in mind that the uses that follow are the tip of the iceberg; the properties of just one oil could fill a book. I've listed the benefits that have helped my clients the most on a daily basis.

— **Lavender:** If I was stranded on a desert island and had to choose only one oil, lavender would be the winner due to its flexibility and gentleness. It's one of the best all-around essential oils, helping bring balance to our emotions and fending off depression, mood swings, and headaches. Lavender has been used in the treatment of depression and insomnia with good results.[6] Every home should have a bottle because of its effectiveness in treating burns and scalds (before attempting to use oils on the skin, check for allergic reactions by testing on a small area). A natural antibiotic, antiseptic, and detoxifier, lavender promotes healing, prevents scarring, and stimulates the immune system. It works its magic by stimulating the cells of a wound to regenerate more quickly, assisting in the healing of insect bites, infections, and other skin issues. (Remember to always dilute essential oils with a carrier oil when applying externally.) One technique that my clients use frequently is placing a few drops of lavender oil on a tissue and tucking it under their pillow as they fall asleep. Many have reported feeling more relaxed and peaceful. In some cases, insomnia symptoms were greatly reduced or eliminated, allowing more restful sleep and greater energy upon waking.

— **Peppermint:** Highly stimulating and refreshing, peppermint is often used in toothpastes and mouthwash to combat bad breath. Perhaps one of the best oils for mental clarity,[7] it perks us up and energizes us for tedious mental tasks. Great for migraines, colds, and respiration, it's also effective for stomach problems such as indigestion. Peppermint helps repel bugs—simply place a few drops on a tissue and tuck it in a pocket before heading out into the woods. Be sure to always keep this oil well away from the eyes when inhaling, because the vapors can cause the eyes to tear. If you're experiencing fatigue, simply inhaling peppermint essential oil helps provide a refreshing burst of energy.

— **Rosemary:** One of the reasons I enjoy this amazing oil is because of its tremendous diversity. Rosemary is a fantastic mental stimulant,[8] and many of my clients keep it on their desks for when they need a quick mental boost at work. They simply inhale the scent for a few breaths and feel invigorated. Rosemary essential oil (diluted with water in a glass spray bottle) is wonderful to spritz around the home in the morning when we're waking up, getting dressed, or brushing our teeth. Inhaling the pleasant aroma helps to mentally energize us for the day ahead. Athletes often add a drop to their lotions to assist sprains and loosen tight muscles (a drop can be added to bathwater, too). Rosemary also works well for depression, fatigue, memory loss, headaches, colds, and flu. Women have reported good results in adding a drop of rosemary to their shampoo for increased hair volume, manageability, and fullness.

— **Thyme:** This powerful antiviral oil posseses antibiotic, antiseptic, and diuretic properties, making it useful for whooping cough, colds, bronchitis, sinus issues, wounds, and the elimination of toxic wastes from the body.[9] Thyme is the first ingredient in the Breathing Easier steam distillation I discuss later in this section. During the summer, the oil can be used as an insect repellent by placing a few drops on a tissue and tucking the tissue in a pocket. Individuals have reported good results using thyme for insomnia by placing a drop on a tissue and putting it under their pillow when going to sleep.

— **Lemon:** One of the most familiar scents, this oil is excellent for use in mental concentration.[10] It stimulates the immune system and is antiviral. People have used lemon essential oil as an antiseptic and antibacterial to help treat insect bites and headaches. The fresh citrus scent invigorates us and encourages extra mental clarity. A drop added to a small glass spray bottle filled with water can serve as a bath and room freshener. Some of my clients have reported good results using lemon essential oil diluted with water for cleaning mirrors and sinks and removing nail polish from floors.

— **Geranium:** This oil is flowery and fragrant (similar to rose). It's a wonderful scent that has profound effects on the emotions. Geranium combats depression and makes a wonderful relaxation oil that can be used during stressful times in an evening bath. It has numerous applications, particularly for all types of skin conditions, and is good for menopausal symptoms, throat infections,[11] wound healing, soothing tight muscles, insomnia, and mental restlessness. It's a good idea to alternate oils every few weeks to maintain optimal effectiveness. If you're using lavender oil under your pillow for several weeks, try alternating with geranium or another soothing oil of choice.

— **Clove:** This oil has been used in toothache treatments for ages. Clove essential oil is highly antiviral and important to have during the winter because it stimulates the immune system and is good for preventing disease and infection.[12] Clove has also been used for digestive problems and muscular disorders. A wonderfully stimulating and revitalizing oil, it can be used when we need a quick mental pick-me-up because it stimulates the brain. Clove should not be used undiluted on the skin.

— **Grapefruit:** This sweet and zesty scent is uplifting and revitalizing for the brain. It's wonderful to inhale when we need additional energy for studying or exercising. Grapefruit essential oil has numerous other uses and helps with bacterial and fungal infections, digestive problems,[13] and depression. Adding a drop to shampoo or lotions helps stimulate the lymphatic system and aids the body in removing excess toxins. If grapefruit oil is not available, simply purchase a grapefruit and save the peels for inhalation during the day as a refreshing energy boost.

— **Ginger:** This works well for headaches, poor memory, diarrhea, and colds and flu.[14] A spicy oil, ginger is frequently used to soothe minor digestive discomforts[15] and increase stamina. This oil has proven to be essential for traveling, especially for those sensitive to motion sickness on boats and planes. Ginger essential oil posses powerful anti-inflammatory properties.[16] It's stimulating to the brain and can be used in the morning or during tedious mental work.

— **Oregano:** Hippocrates praised oregano's benefits for respiratory diseases, ulcers, burns, and poor digestion.[17] This essential oil is a powerful antioxidant,[18] making it a potent ally in protecting cells from free radicals. Mentally stimulating and energizing, it can be inhaled any time during the day to increase cognitive function. Adding a drop to lotions can help ease tense muscles.

Dispersing Delights

My clients have found incredible success in using essential oils diluted with water in small-to-medium glass spray bottles. A few drops of oil mixed with water makes an effective tool that can be misted indoors to freshen the atmosphere. A few quick spritzes around the bedroom when waking up in the morning helps invigorate you and starts the day off on a good note. It's been a blessing for people who decided to give up coffee in the morning. Clients who suffered from insomnia for years found tremendous success with using relaxing oils before bedtime. Simply placing a few drops of lavender or geranium on a cotton ball or facial tissue under the pillow helps you unwind and promotes drifting off to slumberland quickly and soundly.

My clients have enjoyed the following spray mixtures. You can also experiment with combinations that appeal to your individual taste.

DISINFECTANT ROOM SPRAY

1 drop peppermint
1 drop lemon
1 drop rosemary
1 drop clove
2 drops thyme
2 ounces water

Combine ingredients with water in a glass spray bottle (dark glass is best) and shake well before using. Spray away from fabrics, as oils can stain the materials.

MORNING WAKE-ME-UP SPRAY

1 drop lemon
1 drop peppermint
2 drops rosemary
2 drops grapefruit
2 ounces water

Combine ingredients with water in a dark glass spray bottle and shake well. Spray around the room upon waking in the morning or in the bathroom while brushing your teeth.

EVENING RELAXATION SPRAY

3 drops lavender
3 drops geranium
2 ounces water

Combine ingredients with water in a dark glass spray bottle and shake well. Spray around the bed or on a facial tissue to place under your pillow.

Breathing Easier

Respiratory complaints are quite common today and include congestion, runny nose, sinus infections, and cough. Many such ailments are caused by viruses, and essential oils are welcome friends that can help relieve symptoms. Steam is one of the easiest and most effective methods for delivering essential oils to the sinuses and lungs, providing warm, moist air to help open up the nasal and bronchial passages.

BREATHE EASIER STEAM INHALATION

1 drop clove
1 drop oregano
1 drop lavender
2 drops thyme
5–6 cups of water
1 small towel

Boil the water in a pot, turn off the heat, and allow to cool for a few minutes. Pour the water into a bowl and carefully place on a sturdy table. Add the essential oils to the water. Lean over the bowl and use the towel to partially cover your head while breathing in deeply. Keep eyes closed so that they aren't affected. If steaming is not an option (while you're at work or on the road), inhale a tissue scented with the oils.

Enjoy experimenting with your favorite essential oils and appreciate their goodness.

Dimming Artificial Light

Once upon a time, before electricity and automation took over, we lived harmoniously with the cycles of nature. This meant that we woke up with the sun and went to sleep when darkness fell. Not anymore.

The invention of the lightbulb and all the technology since then has created a 24-hour buzz that allows us to work or play all night long. It's not enough to just own houses or cars anymore; numerous cities such as Las Vegas invite us to "own the night" by making entertainment and food available around the clock.

Melatonin is a hormone produced by a tiny structure in our brain called the pineal gland, which is intimately affiliated with the optic system of our eyes. Nighttime darkness signals the gland to release melatonin, making us feel drowsy and relaxed. When we're exposed to bright, artificial lights, however, the process is stopped.

Artificial light wreaks havoc on numerous hormones that are designed to function with the cycles of the sun, not a lightbulb. The body thinks it's daytime when it's really night. This overproduces certain hormones and stops the release of others. We're also more likely to crave sweets for a quick pick-me-up, and stop exercising because of the resulting fatigue.

In the early 1900s, people often slept for more than ten hours per night. Today, we're lucky to get five to seven hours of restful slumber. In the never-ending quest to acquire material possessions and prestige, we're encouraged to sleep less and do more. Physical rest is now considered a waste of valuable time as people turn to coffee, processed sugar, and tobacco to sustain their rest-impoverished lifestyle. Since we're not adequately informed about the subject, we're easily influenced into sacrificing our sleep.

During sleep, a hormonal symphony is orchestrated and performed. The body secretes hormones that help control our appetite, energy metabolism (how many calories we use while at rest), and glucose processing. Not getting enough sleep upsets the balance of the stress hormone cortisol and also affects insulin production, which is important for glucose (blood sugar) regulation and fat storage. Leptin, a hormone that alerts our brain when we've had enough food, is similarly influenced by sleep, along with hormones that stimulate appetite (not something we want if we're looking to lose or maintain weight).

The price we pay for not getting sufficient sleep is incredibly high. Depression, anxiety, exhaustion, weight gain, diabetes, heart disease, and metabolic problems are just some of the problems that can manifest when we abandon this essential component of mental and physical health.

While many of us would greatly benefit from getting back into our natural rhythms, waking up with the sun and going to sleep when darkness falls, most of our modern environments and commitments simply don't allow for this. We may arrive home from work when it's already dark and still have to cook, clean, and care for our family. Without electric light, this would not be possible—or at least not convenient.

What we *can* do is start dimming the lights as we get closer to our relaxation and sleep time. Make sure you can see well enough to avoid tripping or running into objects, but avoid having the house too bright. Lowering the lights and turning off unnecessary lamps will help your body get into sleep mode.

Solving Puzzles in Our Sleep

Today more than ever before, the brain is bombarded continually with facts and figures. Imagine trying to assemble a giant jigsaw puzzle while additional pieces are being thrown at you. It's only when the fragments stop flying that you can step back and try to fit the sections into locations that will allow a full picture to unfold.

Sleep is that vital period when our brain organizes thoughts and ideas and "lays down" memory. The brain is essentially making sense and solving the puzzles of the day as we sleep. While our body may look inert on the bed, the brain is far from dormant—in fact, some brain structures are actually *more* active during sleep than while awake. As we get some shut-eye, the brain consolidates, strengthens, organizes, restructures memories, and "practices" skills we learned while awake.[19]

When new information is introduced to us, the brain acquires and stores the data. As it's consolidated, it becomes more stable and easier to access. At this point, we can recall the information. These steps are all necessary for proper memory function, and this recall consolidation takes place during sleep through the *strengthening of the neural connections* that form our memories.[20] Without proper rest, these neurons don't fire optimally. This is why newborns and infants sleep constantly. Their brains are growing and developing; all data provided to them is fresh, and they need the additional time to assimilate the new information into their brain neurons.

Losing only a few hours of sleep per night can impair our ability to think and function because even *one* shortened sleep cycle initiates a stress response in the body. Lack of rest undermines the immune system and makes us more vulnerable to colds, influenza, and other diseases. In addition, it impairs our reflexes and decision-making skills. The more physical challenges we have, whether due to stress or illness, the more rest the body requires to recuperate and repair itself.

Sufficient rest and sleep are just as critical as a proper diet and should not be discounted just because of the unfounded promptings of others who encourage us to work long hours. Physical exercise, strenuous and tedious mental work, and worry all play a role in adding to our rest requirements.

We Snooze, We Win

You may have heard the saying, "You snooze, you lose," but I hope the preceding information helped you to think differently. When you make rest one of your priorities, you can begin to gain the benefits of greater cognitive functioning and physical health. Remember, sufficient sleep improves moods, enhances learning, helps regulate the appetite, improves memory, and so much more. Take a look at the following tips about getting sufficient sleep and enjoy the benefits of essential rest.

Tips for Restful Sleep

- Limit TV before going to sleep. Shutting off the television even one hour before bed is challenging for most people because many programs and commercials exert a hypnotic and stimulating effect on the brain. Start by muting the sound during commercials and try lowering the volume as you get closer to bedtime.

- Wait until you feel tired to get into bed. If you're feeling too energetic, you'll be more apt to toss and turn when you try to fall asleep. This can lead to feelings of frustration, especially if you start to glance at the clock and count how many hours you have left until the alarm goes off.

- Try to wind down at least one hour before going to bed. Listen to relaxing music, enjoy a warm bath, and slow down.

- Avoid being online before going to sleep. Computer headlines keep us stimulated and curious to find out the latest news. Turn the computer off at least an hour before bed and focus on relaxing activities.

- Turn the lights down an hour before bedtime. Dimming the lights helps signal that it's time to wind down for the day. The brain counts on these cues to release hormones that relax us.

- Listen to soothing music. Try to avoid fast-paced, loud songs that stimulate the body into moving. Focus instead on mellow tunes that relax the mind.

- Try to get to get to sleep before 10 P.M. or as far ahead of midnight as possible. This may be the most challenging suggestion, but try it to see how it makes you feel. The increase in energy should be noticeable.

- Practice going to bed and waking up around the same time every day, even on weekends. We often try to "catch up" on Saturday and Sunday, but this can make us more tired during the week. Try to follow a routine whenever possible.

- Make space in the day for activities that cause physical exertion. Moving enough helps the body release excess energy, which makes falling asleep easier.

- Use relaxing aromatherapy smells around the bedtime such as lavender and orange to increase relaxation levels. Simply place a few drop of your favorite relaxing essential oils on a tissue and tuck under your pillow.

The brain-enhancing tools you now possess will help keep your magnificent superstructure functioning at its best. Keep focusing on including brain-building foods and spices in your diet; challenge your brain with unique, expansive thinking; enjoy positive music and delightful essential oils; and allow your mind and body to recharge and rejuvenate with sufficient rest. In the next chapter, you'll learn why movement is critical for our well-being, including our mind.

Part III

THE PILLAR
OF MOTION

CHAPTER 7

INTRODUCING FUN TO MOVEMENT

The laborsaving devices the Industrial Revolution introduced brought welcome relief to our great-grandparents. As a result, we now possess technological marvels that make human motion almost unnecessary. While electricity and automation helped us to control the environment, they have also injured us by discouraging natural body movement.

Putting motion on the back burner has resulted in devastating consequences, not only physically, but also for our mental and emotional stability. We've invited an increase in diabetes, obesity, heart disease, high blood pressure, cognitive decline, and postural abnormalities due to the influence of a sedentary existence.

Our cultural momentum has steadily shifted us toward inactive lifestyles filled with excessive digital stimulation, lack of movement, and insufficient quality rest. Laborsaving devices heist physical movements out of our day, discouraging key primal motions necessary for optimal body functioning such as bending, reaching, walking, twisting, pulling, and squatting. Frequent dining out means we seldom even shop for our food (push a cart, reach, squat, bend down, carry bags), work at washing and chopping produce, or clean up after we're done. These seemingly small deprivations of movement add up over time, magnifying the cumulative negative effects on our health. For many years, I've witnessed firsthand how harmful a motionless lifestyle is to mental and physical well-being—it's nothing short of a physiological and emotional disaster.

The typical day in the life of an average working person lacks not only sunshine and fresh air, but also general fun and essential movement. Many of us wake up in the morning after sleeping for seven to eight hours without motion. During breakfast, we're sitting again without much activity. Then we continue being sedentary by sitting in a car or bus on our way to work. We finally arrive at the office for another eight hours of dormant sitting without much motion. At the end of the workday, it's the same process, except the sitting destination is now the couch. We repeat this routine for days, months, and finally decades. As time passes, we wonder why we feel weaker, stiffer, and more imbalanced.

As little as 100 years ago, our current sedentary lifestyle was unheard of. In the past, farmers and other laborers worked from morning until evening. Waking early, people toiled in the fields and returned home when darkness fell. Hearing the phrase, "Sweetheart, I need to get a workout in before we eat dinner," was simply impossible because the whole day was a workout! Individuals "exercised" all day long by moving their bodies continually.

Today, we've become a nation of sedentary multitasking experts. Every second of the day is jam-packed. We're watching TV, talking on the phone, texting, surfing the Internet, eating, and answering our kids' questions—all at the same time. While we *do more,* we *move less,* to our detriment.

Why We Need Motion

A healthy body is supple, strong, and agile, with balance and good cognitive function well into later years. It's up to us to provide essential physical movement to stimulate our immune and respiratory systems and to build proper bone density.

Motion helps release endorphins, the natural substances that reduce pain and promote feelings of euphoria. Vigorous movement causes a rise in temperature, which can help inhibit bacterial and viral growth in the body.[1] Increased respiration helps clear our lungs of germs, delivering more oxygen to lung tissue.

Physical exertion pumps oxygen into the heart and throughout the body and causes the expansion of blood vessels and arteries, which allows blood to move more efficiently and freely. Movement keeps us digesting and absorbing our food and assists the lymphatic system in destroying unwanted pathogens.[2] One of the challenges we face is a low-functioning and compromised immune system, and lack of motion is a part of the problem.

Optimal brain functioning requires movement for increased circulation, delivery of vital oxygen, and the formation of new blood vessels. Movement improves oxygen circulation through the brain, which sharpens our thinking, boosts our moods, reduces stress and anxiety,[3] and stimulates regions of the brain involved in learning and memory.[4]

Our bodies flourish with sufficient motion and waste away with disuse. If we challenge them, we improve, and in turn we're rewarded with greater flexibility, coordination, and strength; clearer thinking; happier moods; and a more joyous attitude.

Where's the Fun?

If we glance inside a large fitness facility today, we'll see patrons *sitting* on stationary bicycles while reading magazines and others walking on treadmills while watching television. Many large health clubs have more TVs than electronics stores.

The attraction to reading and watching TV while exercising should offer us valuable information, namely that these motions are not engaging our minds (boring) and feel like drudgery. Also, the movements are repetitive and eventually become unchallenging, both physiologically and mentally. Being distracted with outside stimulation helps the time "go by faster."

When we enter a club to "work out" on the quest to counteract our sedentary lifestyle, we place ourselves in a closed environment that lacks sunshine and fresh air. Many weight machines require us to sit or lie down, mimicking the common postures of our daily routines.

How many times have we seen drivers looking for a closer parking space at the gym, only to walk in the door and step on a treadmill? To our detriment, we begin to see specific locations as places where we move our bodies and, as a result, miss out on the countless daily opportunities to engage in beneficial physical motions.

Isn't it interesting that we build machines that stop us from moving, like remote controls, riding lawn mowers, dishwashers, cars, and escalators, and then build machines that force us to move, such as treadmills and stationary bikes? I believe we should just cut out the intermediary and do many activities ourselves. Most of our motion should come from daily life, not 30 minutes in a gym.

What we're missing most in traditional exercise routines is the *fun* component. We're not playing enough—or at all—while moving our bodies, and this lack of joy encourages us to avoid motion, to our own disservice. If you think of movement as difficult and boring, you won't be motivated to get off the couch. But if you start incorporating games and having fun, you'll stick with it forever because these aspects will inspire you to come back for more.

When we combine *fun* and *laughter* with movement, we gain profound health benefits emotionally, physically, and psychologically. New clients often look to me for permission to have fun. They believe they're not supposed to enjoy moving their bodies—and if they do, then it can't be good for them—but the opposite is true. When we feel good, it's a strong indicator we're doing something right. Enjoyment is a form of positive communication with ourselves.

Start visualizing fun as oxygen, as a necessity. It's when we stop playing that our lives begin to seem empty and dull, and we lose the ability to feel deep joy. Begin to view fun and play as the remedies that help us stay emotionally, mentally, and physically exuberant.

Humans thrive on discovering; it's one of the ways we learn and retain information in an effective and efficient manner. Our brains are naturally hardwired to engage in joyous play because it reduces stress, brings out laughter and creativity, and creates spontaneity. It also helps us bond with others socially. We learn more about ourselves and become open to creative possibilities.[5] I believe that play is just as vital to our well-being as restful sleep and healthy food. It keeps us feeling good and inspires us to move, and this combination is a winning recipe that leads to consistency, real enjoyment, and positive health benefits.

It's a shame that our society frowns on playing once we reach adulthood. Humans play as children, but as we age, we're encouraged to put away the toys, grab a briefcase, and join the "real" world. Many adults feel guilty when they play because they've been taught that it's a waste of time. When was the last time you had a belly laugh? If you can't remember, it's an indicator that play isn't a frequent part of your day. Adults spend too little time at play and could benefit from it the most. Slowly, workplaces are starting to learn that playing on the job leads to more productivity, bonding, creativity, energy, enthusiasm, and greater problem solving, and I hope this trend continues.

The Miraculous Power of Play

Tom's parents brought him to my office because he was suffering from obesity and low self-esteem. Not quite a teenager, he was already more than 200 pounds. The extra weight made Tom feel self-conscious and depressed, and his parents hoped that I could help improve his health and confidence.

When I first met Tom, his head was down and he barely spoke. Halfway through our session, he continued to resist fully communicating and still looked despondent. Because *playful motion creates joyful emotions,* I decided to bring in some fun movement.

I took a balloon, quickly inflated it, and asked Tom if he would hit it back and forth with me in the hallway. When the boy looked at the brightly colored balloon, his eyes took on a sparkle and his posture became more alert. As I tossed it to him, his demeanor changed. He started smiling, hitting the balloon back and forth with me, and visibly relaxed.

As we tapped the balloon to each other, sometimes missing, sometimes connecting, I witnessed an amazing metamorphosis: Tom began to goof around, play, and communicate. He started to open up and express himself more. I helped him anchor movement with the fun he was having so that his brain could associate motion with positive, joyous feelings. This would inspire him to look for ways to add more movement into his life—not because he had to, but because he wanted to have fun. In just this short session, Tom transformed before my eyes from feeling depressed and lethargic to being an energetic person filled with joyous laughter. It was the beginning of his regained confidence, and it all started with the inspiring power of play.

I've seen numerous miracles when using play as a powerful catalyst for fun physical movement. When I provided geriatric classes on balance and coordination skills, seniors would often walk in lethargic, depressed, and tired. All of that quickly changed when I turned on the industrial-strength bubble maker that I'd brought along. I placed the machine on a large table with wheels and turned on some fast-paced music. Each senior received a set of chopsticks with the goal of catching as many bubbles as possible.

Soon, cascades of sparkling bubbles filled the air as I pushed the magical device around the room. The seniors quickly perked up and become exuberant. They began laughing while reaching and bending to try to catch the moving bubbles; expressing delight, amusement, and joy, much like children. The energy in the room took on a euphoric life of its own, causing people passing by in the hallway to pause, glance in, and start to laugh just from watching the fun.

Joy is contagious. Seeing others experience this emotion influences us to feel it, too, even if we're not actively engaged in the activity. Many seniors would specifically ask to have the magical bubble machine back for an encore, looking forward to enjoying it again. This is one of the key elements of fun—it keeps us coming back!

Ways to Incorporate More Fun and Motion

Movement keeps our muscles and mind vigorous, childlike, curious, playful, excited, and happy. All we have to do is become more conscious of providing this valuable resource to ourselves *more* throughout the day. Take a look at the following suggestions for bringing more joyous motion into your routine.

- Moving the body while listening to engaging music often leads to dancing. This is one of the most fun and most creative activities because we're inspired by the music to make up movements. Explore joining dance classes or groups that teach unfamiliar steps. Try salsa, flamenco, disco, hip-hop, break dancing, and ballet. Leave all apprehensions at the door, let go, and have fun trying something new. Practice dancing at home to different musical styles. Release all self-consciousness and move the body freely.

- Enjoy nature by hiking outdoors. Being close to the earth, smelling the vegetation, looking for birds and small animals, and taking the time to listen to the sounds of the environment are all health-promoting activities. Kids often spend much of their time indoors, and taking them outside to look at plants and insects is one of the best educational experiences they can enjoy. Encourage children to be aware of their environment and learn how to respect our planet.

- Bicycling outdoors is popular and fun. It's one of the best activities because almost anyone can engage in it regardless of fitness level. Invite friends and family to go bike riding, discover the landscape, and enjoy being outside.

- If you enjoy watching sports like baseball, chances are you'll enjoy playing them as well. Look for leagues to join in the area or invite neighbors, family members, and friends to a game in the park. You don't have to be a pro. The goal is to just have fun and encourage others to do the same.

- While kids are naturally open to play, we need to be especially diligent in encouraging our elderly population to engage in fun activity because they not only move the least, but need it the most for enhanced brain function, circulation, and memory, and to combat depression and lethargy.

- We often save our playfulness for when we leave on vacation and, as a result, end up having fun only two weeks out of the year. Take some time every day to engage in a mini-vacation. Visit a spa, prepare a fancy meal, give your hands or feet a massage, and try a beauty treatment such as a mud mask for the face or leave-in conditioner for the hair. Pampering ourselves is fun and it increases our self-esteem.

- Actively seek out activities that encourage smiling and laughter. Make up games by using creativity and imagination every day. Look for people genuinely interested in having fun for its own sake and who possess a playful nature. These people often appear young or childlike regardless of their age.

- Fun fitness equipment can keep us interested and motivated to try new motions. Great examples are medicine balls, exercise bands, hand weights, kettle bells, and agility ladders. Make up movements or use makeshift items in the home. Cans of beans can be used as small hand weights; putting your feet on the couch while doing a push-up will challenge your body more. Experiment, using your creativity and imagination.

- Our facial muscles need the motion of smiling. It automatically releases feel-good chemicals in the brain, even if we believe that we have nothing or no one to smile at. Just as we need to stretch our legs after sitting for long periods of time, we need to stretch our facial muscles. Often, people's expressions freeze into frowns or scowls. Let the smile lines on your face show the happiness and laughter you've experienced.

- If you take care of a dog, daily walks can turn into opportunities to play and chase one another. Bring a ball to the park to throw and run around.

- Cleaning the house is a great physical activity that encourages bending, twisting, reaching, and squatting. The movements leave our home looking better, which helps us feel more organized, joyful, and at peace.

- Doing yard work engages the whole body while we enjoy the fresh air and sunshine. Creating a visually appealing natural environment right outside our door brings out creativity and fun. Encouraging family members and friends to rake leaves with us builds a sense of togetherness. Being close to nature and appreciating the trees, leaves, and grass enhances our well-being.

- If you keep procrastinating having fun, playing, or waiting to move more until you're not as busy, chances are you'll never do it. By the time we reach our later years, many of us lose much of the ability to have fun, along with our health. Make it a priority to play and move today. It's that important.

Daily Movement Questions

- Did I move my body from head to toe today?
- Did I often smile genuinely?
- Did I live an active life?
- Are the people I'm spending time with daily inspiring me to frown or smile?
- Did I move my hands and feet frequently (not just to type on a keyboard or press the car gas pedal)?

- Did I make my immediate environment more conducive to motion? (Some examples include hiding the remote control, getting up off the couch to change the channel, and walking to get a drink of water instead of asking someone to bring it to you.)

- Am I engaging in physical activities that promote fun and laughter throughout the day?

- Did I make it a point to bring play into my life today?

Look for motion that contributes to something fun and engaging. *The secret is to sneak motion in throughout the day and make it almost unnoticeable.* It's the *frequency* that makes it so effective. This only requires a series of *small adjustments* that add up to big *improvements.*

Greater health leads to increased happiness, which overflows to everyone. Imagine the transformative effect we'll automatically have on loved ones by filling our lives with motion. The many different movements described in this book will help guide everyone toward more fun. The point is to get moving and do it often. We're designed to experience joy, and motion leads the way.

So Many Motions, So Little Time

Sometimes schedules can get so busy that we stop getting the movement we need to keep us functioning at our best. We may have the best intentions and try hard to make the time, but circumstances beyond our control can make finding even 15 consecutive minutes almost impossible.

We know how important motion is for well-being and how great we feel when we experience it. The challenge is to fit it in consistently. Luckily, we can sneak fitness into our life all day long using short, 30-second to one-minute increments.

Our bodies see all movement as a positive investment of time. It's a *cumulative* process. To the body, *any investment in movement is a benefit.* This means we can accomplish an amazing all-day workout just by sneaking in a few minutes of motion here and there.

Take a look at the following photos for ideas about how to sneak movement into the day and explore the various movement and fitness modalities in the coming sections.

Side Planks

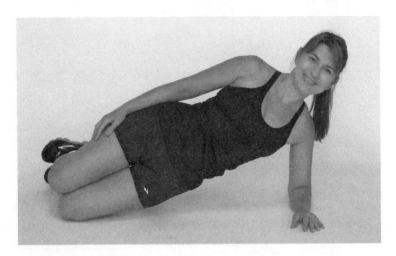

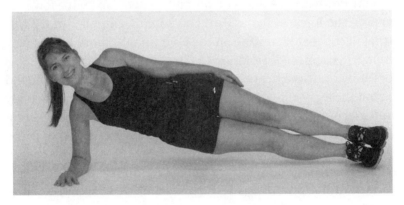

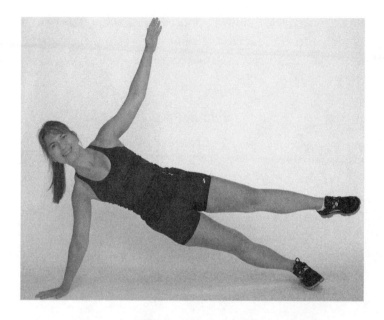

A side plank is one of the quickest and most effective motions we can sneak into our day. It doesn't require equipment or much space, and it can be modified to challenge all fitness levels. Begin by lying down on one side. Lift your upper body up on the forearm, keeping the forearm flat against the floor. Beginners can try this with knees bent and resting on the floor initially, until greater core strength is achieved. Hold for 15–30 seconds. Alternate sides. As core and arm strength are increased, lift the knees off the floor and extend the legs parallel with the floor. Hold the weight of the body on the arm closest to the floor. Work up to holding the position for 15–30 seconds or longer. When these movements become too easy, hold your body up on one hand, using the wrist for support, extend the opposite arm toward the ceiling, and raise the same side leg toward the sky. This is an advanced movement and requires time to build up to.

Partner-Plank Balloon Game

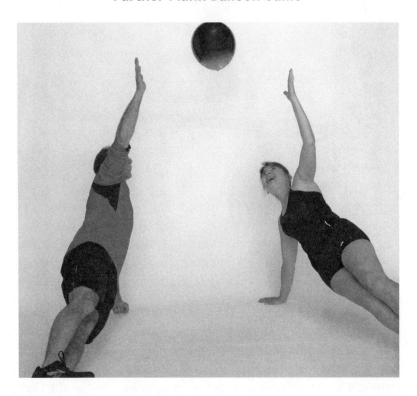

Blow up a balloon and perform a plank several feet across from a partner. Tap the balloon to one another while holding a plank. If a partner isn't available, tap the balloon against the wall. This is an excellent drill for training core strength and reflexes. Kids love this activity because it's fun and engaging.

Partner Rope Pull

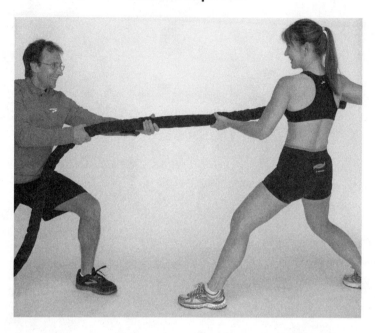

Sneak in pulling motions during the day by grabbing a sturdy rope or rolled towel and trying to pull it back and forth with a partner. This movement engages numerous muscles in the body, and making a game out of it enhances the fun. Use caution in case your partner lets go of the rope.

Just imagine what making small additions of movements could do to your muscle tone, circulation, stamina, and self-esteem. When you make time for motion during the day, you affirm that your health and well-being are important, and you build your confidence. Even if you couldn't find another minute to visit a gym or take a walk, you'd still feel good that you accomplished some fun and challenging motions.

CHAPTER 8
PLAYING WITH MOTIONS

One of the reasons my clients love the workouts I challenge them with is because they're fun and engaging not only to the body, but also to the mind. Clients tell me that their workout sessions are joyous because they're playing and getting in shape instead of doing boring exercises. It's common for them to laugh so hard that they have to stop moving for a moment.

In the following sections, I'll share some of my favorite tools, techniques, and equipment to encourage you to incorporate some of these modalities into your daily motion practice. We're all unique and special, and some ideas will appeal to you more than others. Exploring these motions will encourage you to keep coming back to moving the body consistently. Remember to use your creativity to make up exercises that are fun and challenging to you. Listen to your body for feedback and enjoy the health benefits of your increased fitness.

Skipping to Health

When we think of jumping rope, it usually brings back memories of playing as a kid. For many, that was the last time we engaged in this fun activity. That's really a shame because jumping rope isn't just for children. Adding this enjoyable practice to our movement routine can be one of the most effective, efficient, and fun ways to attain great physical and cardiovascular fitness.

Jumping rope, also called skipping, is an amazing full-body workout that engages our legs, arms, core, and cardiovascular system. As we jump, the brain is challenged to make extremely quick calculations in judging the rope's distance, direction, speed, and position. Skipping combines rhythm and timing, and challenges us to make fast decisions that help build body coordination and balance.

This movement can help provide protection against osteoporosis because it's a weight-bearing activity; every time we land on our feet, stress force is applied to the skeletal system, helping us to develop and maintain much needed bone mass.[1] Jumping rope is one of the best training modalities used by many athletes in numerous sports because it helps improve reflexes—the ability to physically react quickly and easily to a given challenge.

What's great about skipping is everyone can be involved and included. Kids love to see adults jumping, and it sets a good example for keeping them fit in the future. Some people avoid jumping rope because their arms and legs are out of tune from lack of practice, and this can cause the rope to get caught under their feet. It can be frustrating and irritating if the rope gets tangled or hits the body. This is one of the reasons I added a unique spin by cutting the jump rope in half, creating two pieces that everyone can use to simulate skipping and avoid these frustrating situations. The movements are similar to regular skipping, except we no longer become ensnared in the rope. We receive all the great benefits without a snag!

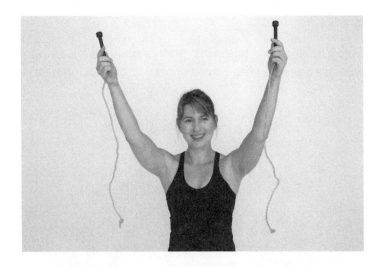

It's easy to take a jump rope with you when you're traveling because it's small, lightweight, portable, and easy to fit into a purse or small bag. You can accomplish a great workout in a hotel room or, if you have access to a playground or a park outside, you can take advantage of it and get some fresh air and sunshine.

Jumping rope burns a tremendous amount of calories in a very short time and doesn't have to be done all at once to gain the benefits. One method of training includes lifting some weights or doing body-weight exercises and working in several minutes of skipping rope in between repetitions. The key is to always switch the patterns of jumping to make it more fun and exciting. You can use your creativity to make up countless foot arrangements. Remember to rotate the rope forward so there's less chance of hitting your face or eyes. Also, try skipping on one leg at a time and then the other. Start out slow and increase both the time and speed.

Jump-Rope Variations

Take a look at the following photos for inspiration on some footwork patterns that can be incorporated into a skipping routine.

Feet Together, Feet Apart

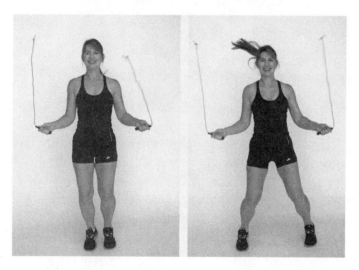

Jump rope while moving the feet together and apart.

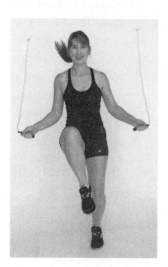

Alternating High Knees

Alternate lifting the knees, or keep one knee lifted for a count of ten then shift to the opposite knee for a count of ten.

Side-to-Side Toe Tap

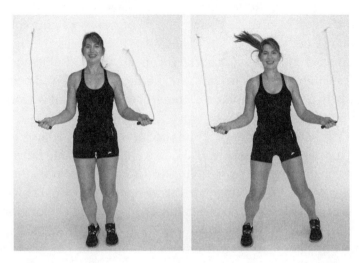

Alternate tapping the foot to the side, taking turns with each leg or tapping one foot out for a count of ten and switching to the other foot.

Bands for Resilience

Exercise bands and tubes are some of the simplest and most effective gear I use and recommend. The body doesn't know the difference between lifting a weight and moving against resistance; it just knows there's muscular tension and responds accordingly by getting stronger. Bands or tubes come in different colors, which represent different levels of tension. The higher rigidity is accomplished by making the bands thicker, providing a greater challenge.

Bands can be used with a partner or alone, and the combinations of motions are limitless. Working out with a partner can help increase our motivation and consistency, and bands are perfect partner tools because each person can enjoy a workout at the same time.

Everyone from beginners to accomplished athletes can benefit by incorporating resistance bands and tubes in their fitness program because they add fun and variety, and are convenient and affordable. Bands are somewhat safer than weights since there's no risk of injury from dropping heavy dumbbells on feet. They don't require a spotter because there's no risk of heavy weights collapsing on the body. They're also quiet, allowing us to easily sneak in a great workout without waking anyone in the house. Bands and tubes are light, are easy to carry, and fit into most bags and pockets. They help us build endurance, strength, and power, all within the confines of a small space.

It's wise to vary your programs because the body adjusts to the same motions fairly quickly. If you're working the same range and angle constantly, you cease taxing yourself, become too efficient, and stop seeing improvement. It's also important to avoid boredom and stay consistent, and bands allow creativity and exploration in designing actions unique to your goals. By shortening or lengthening our bands, we gain immediate control of tension levels. Their versatility is enormous because they can be attached to solid anchors, and we can even step on them.

The freedom of movement and greater range of motion is vastly different from machines that control where we start and stop. The bands allow us to create resistance from all directions and mimic the actions we perform in daily life. They can be useful aids in physical therapy, and people in wheelchairs or who otherwise have limited mobility find them to be effective and practical.

Movements with Exercise Bands

Take a look at the following pictures and descriptions. These are some of the ways bands can used to work the chest, triceps, biceps, shoulders, and legs. Be creative by coming up with new movement ideas.

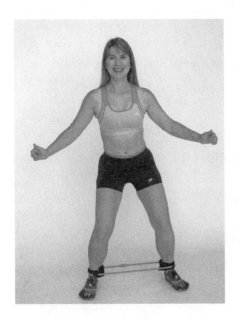

Sideways Walk

Walking sideways with a band around the ankles helps strengthen the legs and gluteus. Try walking for 5–10 steps to the right, then walk 5–10 steps to the left. The legs and gluteus should feel challenged. Since we spend most of the day moving forward, we need side-to-side motions to help balance our leg movement ability.

Standing Row

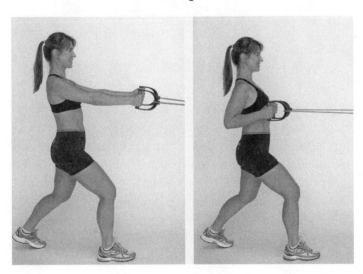

Have a partner hold the band or anchor it around a stable object and grip the handles securely. Face your partner or anchor so that the bands are directly in front of your body. Step back, feeling the band tense, and begin to pull the handles toward the rib cage, thumbs facing the ceiling. Keep the elbows close to the body. The back muscles will be active along with the arms. Work up to 10 repetitions. If this feels too easy, step farther back, increasing the tension of the band, or try a thicker band.

Biceps Curl

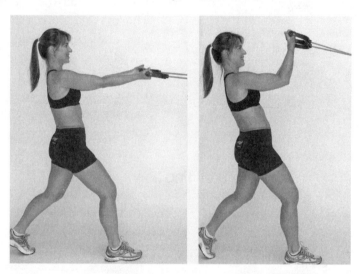

Secure the band around a steady object or have a partner hold the middle of the band. Grip the handles firmly and step backward, creating tension in the band. Lift the palms so that they face the ceiling and hold them parallel to the floor. Imagine the elbows resting on a high table and try to maintain this elbow position throughout the movement. Lift the arms toward the chin, feeling the biceps and core working. Slowly extend the arms back to the starting position, being conscious of keeping the elbows up, as if they're still resting on an imaginary high table. Work toward 10 repetitions. If the movement feels too easy, step farther back to create more band tension or try a thicker band.

Triceps Press

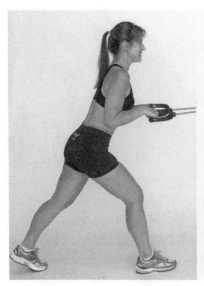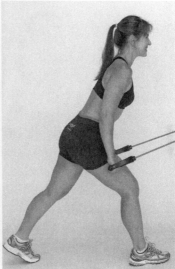

Attach the band securely around a stable object or have a part-ner hold the middle of the band. Grip the handles firmly while positioning the palms to face the floor. Keeping the elbows close to the body, start with the arms in front of the chest and press back toward the hips. Feel the triceps contract and increase the tension of the band by stepping back if needed, or try a thicker band. Work toward 10 repetitions.

Chest Press

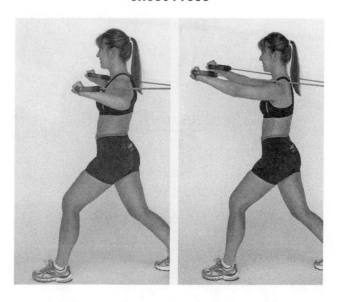

Secure the band around a solid object or have a partner hold the middle of the band. Start with the band behind the body while you face away from your partner or the anchoring object, and grip both handles securely. Step forward to build tension. Press the band in front of the body with both arms simultaneously, at chest level, keeping the palms facing down. You should feel the arms and chest working. Increase the tension by stepping farther forward if needed or try a thicker band. Work toward 5–10 repetitions.

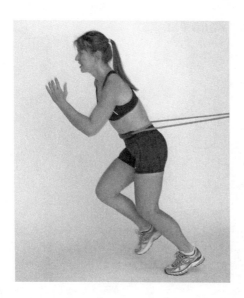

Band Running

Wrap the band around your waist and have a partner hold the handles firmly. Start to slowly move forward while communicating to your partner the tension level necessary for challenging forward motion. Work up to slowly running. This should feel as though you're running through water or molasses. Practice running sideways and backward slowly, while building cardiovascular fitness and strength. Check the band for any damage to avoid breakage. Be cautious with these movements as the band may potentially tear in half or your partner could let go unexpectedly. Work up to running for 15- to 30-second sprints.

Partner Band Planks

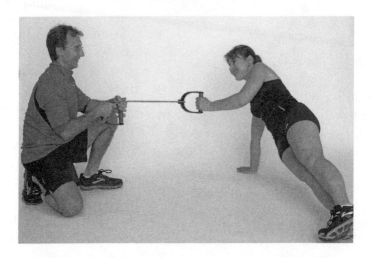

Lie down sideways on the floor facing your partner. Gently lift your body weight on one arm while balancing the body on the extended arm and legs. If this is too difficult, keep both knees on the floor. Firmly grip the band handle with the top free hand in front of the body while your partner also holds the band securely. Pull the band toward your body while keeping the base arm strong. Feel the challenge in the core and arms. Work up to 10 repetitions and alternate sides.

The Missing Link: Balance

The majority of fitness routines today focus primarily on weight loss, endurance, or muscle building, placing balance training last on the list. Since many of us experience a sedentary existence, when we try to fit some maintenance movement into the day, it's frequently walking or jogging on a treadmill, or using weight machines.

Balance is often ignored because we're so focused on our appearance. We forget that balance is necessary for fall and injury prevention,[2] cognitive stimulation, and all-around health. We're under the impression that this type of work is something only gymnasts or acrobats need, and we fail to see its value.

The body is always looking to find a state of equilibrium. There's constant communication between our brain and muscles. These ongoing internal messages allow us to remain stable by sensing our position in space. Balance is partially controlled by the nervous system, so practicing movements that challenge equilibrium helps keep our mind-body connection sharp.

Falls are the leading cause of injury and death among people 65 years of age or older.[3] Regardless of age, it's quite easy for anyone to slip on wet, icy pavement, trip on just about anything, or miss a step on uneven surfaces. When we begin to feel ourselves falling, it's crucial to be able to regain our balance quickly to avoid a potential injury.

The body works as a whole structure. It's sensitive to the countless signals we receive every moment (whether from our feet and toes or what we're seeing with our eyes); and all those signals communicate with our brain, muscles, and nervous system. The body then reacts by making active or inactive the muscles needed to maintain a stable position. We do this every time we get up from a chair, walk, ride a bike, and stand on our tiptoes to grab something from a high shelf. When the body becomes overloaded with information that's too complicated, we have a tendency to lose our balance.

If we begin to practice unusual motions that test us in many different situations, we can increase our ability to recognize challenging stimuli and respond with a better reaction. With training, we can dramatically improve our balance and keep it well into our later years.[4]

The key is putting ourselves off balance in controlled and safe environments. I don't recommend starting instability training on high balance beams where falls can lead to injury. It's best to start slow and build up from there. The good news is that the training is not only easy, it's a great deal of fun and doesn't have to take additional time out of the day.

If you enjoy participating in sports, balance training will enhance your performance by helping you control your body's center of gravity and increasing your efficiency in movement. Practice training on uneven surfaces such as fitness air cushions (the

Bosu balance trainer is one popular brand) and thick ropes placed on the floor. The goal is to train the body to respond to constantly changing surfaces, forces, and elements.

Kids love balance training, too, and it's actually crucial to involve children in balance work because their center of gravity changes as they grow, making their movements seem clumsy and less coordinated. It's easy to see balance improvements quickly as the body adjusts to various situations and challenges. Take a look at the ideas that follow for inspiration on incorporating more balance work in your day. Challenge workout partners, kids, and friends to come up with balance drills as games. This also helps stimulate the mind and enhances problem-solving skills.

Balance Challenges

Balance During Brushing

One of the quickest ways to begin balance training is to stand on one leg as you're brushing your teeth. (Please be cautious about practicing balance drills in the bathroom, as there's no soft padding to help absorb an impact if you fall.) Alternate legs and notice which one has better balance. Work the challenged leg more often and for longer periods of time. Too easy? Close one of your eyes when you're brushing your teeth and standing on one leg, and gradually work up to closing both eyes. It's much more difficult. Feel the body and gauge how it automatically seeks to keep itself upright.

The entire family can make a game out of who can stand on one leg longer while brushing their teeth and keeping their eyes closed. Everyone is usually laughing by the end of the game. As this becomes too easy, simply add another element, like standing on tiptoes, and later incorporate the opposite arm by extending it sideways or above the head. This is great training for body perception.

Towel Balance Challenge

This is one of the best balance drills for putting a smile on both parents' and children's faces. Grab any towel and have two people hold opposite ends while facing one another. Both parties will stand on one foot. Now they'll each pull the towel gently and try to maneuver the other person off balance. Feel free to hop around or just stand in one spot and make a game of it. Whoever has to place the raised foot down to regain their balance needs to do a jumping jack or push-up. This can be played at home or outside, using a jump rope or any sturdy rope instead of a towel.

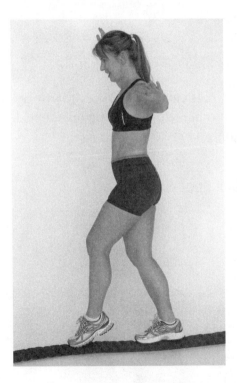

Floor Rope Walk

Walking on a thick rope laid on the floor is a great way to challenge your balance. Extend the arms to the side if necessary, or place the rope close to a wall for additional balance support. Try wearing minimalist shoes such as Vibram FiveFingers, or walk on the rope barefoot (depending on the condition of the rope).

Partner-Balance Rope Drills

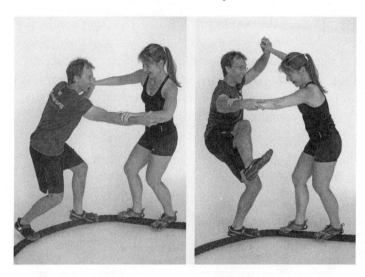

Invite friends and family to participate in balance drills by trying to gently unbalance one another while standing on a rope. If it becomes too easy, try closing your eyes.

Fitness-Ball Knee Balance

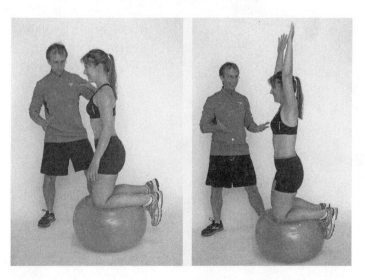

Practice kneeling on a fitness ball (such as a Swiss ball) with the help of a partner or a wall and maintain the position while lifting your arms over your head. Feel the challenge in your core as your body works to remain stable. As this becomes easier, try closing your eyes. This is an advanced exercise and should be practiced with a spotter.

Partner Weighted-Ball Balance Game

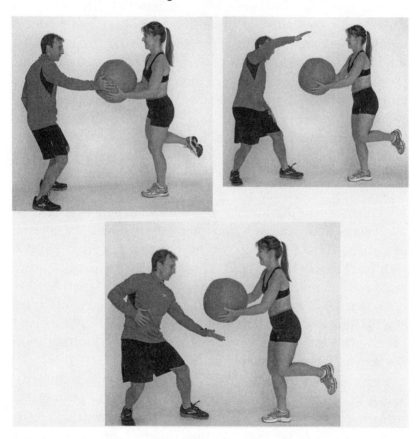

Stand on one foot and hold a medicine ball or similar weighted ball. Face your partner and allow them to gently try to push the ball out of your hands from different angles while you hold on to the ball and maintain your balance. Have your partner push the ball from the top, from the sides, and from underneath. Feel the challenge in both arms, the standing leg, and the core. This helps develop balance, core engagement, and arm strength.

Having a Ball

Medicine-ball training is one of the oldest forms of body conditioning. In ancient Greece, Hippocrates used balls sewn and stuffed with sand. His patients threw them back and forth for injury prevention, hence the name "medicine ball."[5] Even though these tools have been used for centuries, they've gained enormous popularity in recent years, making more people aware of their time-tested benefits. Since they're portable, they can be used practically anywhere: at home, at the beach, outdoors, or while traveling. They're suitable for all ages and fitness levels, easier to use than dumbbells, and provide a universally friendlier version of weight lifting because they're easier on the hands and fingers (a firm grip is needed for dumbbells).

Unlike weight machines, which force us to perform restricted movements, medicine balls don't limit us to using a single plane of motion. This allows us to play in ways that just aren't possible with machines or free weights. We can challenge specific muscle groups or use more than one group at a time.

When a ball is thrown or caught, the path it travels is never exactly the same. We catch it in a unique space every time and engage different muscles for balance and control. This helps train the body to react faster and builds better reflexes.

A big challenge with aging is not just the loss of strength, muscle mass, and bone density, but the loss of power—how quickly we can apply force. Throwing weighted balls allows us to learn how to transfer our momentum from different angles so that our strength, balance, and coordination increases.[6]

Many conditioning programs include impact training such as sprinting, jogging, or step aerobics. However, some people are unable to perform these activities due to a variety of physical limitations.

The medicine ball becomes a crucial element that increases cardio-vascular capacity, builds strength, and improves muscle stamina all at once, without exerting heavy stress on the lower extremities.

Most of us are one-side dominant—that is, we favor one side of our body over the other and consequently develop strength, coordination, and balance challenges as a result. Training with weighted-ball drills can help build strength and flexibility on our non-dominant side. We can replicate the motions of swinging, throwing, and rotating. Many athletes have benefited by incorporating medicine-ball training as a performance-enhancement technique.[7]

In more than two decades of working with athletes and clients, I've been able to successfully use medicine balls with everyone. Over-weight clients (some exceeding 300 pounds), athletes, children with learning challenges, and seniors well into their 90s all had fun and experienced benefits. Try the following motions or create your own. My clients enjoy the weighted balls made by Ugi and Dynamax.

Weighted-Ball Movements

Body Crossover

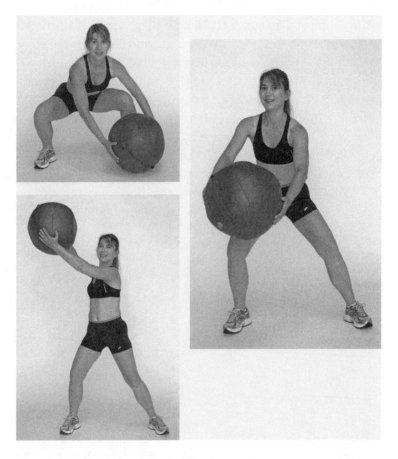

Start with the weighted ball on the floor while keeping the feet shoulder-width apart. Position the ball in front of the left leg. Gently squat down to pick up the ball using the legs while engaging the core. Slowly lift the ball across the body toward the ceiling as if drawing one stroke of the letter X. Return to the starting position following the same line, bringing the ball back to the starting foot. Feel the challenge in the core, legs, and arms. Work up to 10 repetitions and alternate sides.

Whole-Body Engager

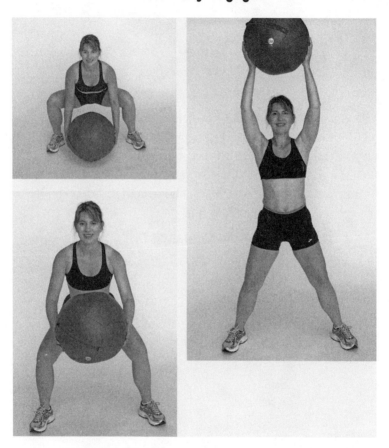

   Place a weighted ball in front of the body and gently squat to pick it up. Slowly lift the ball up over your head, and then bring back down to starting position in a controlled manner. Feel the challenge in the legs, core, and arms. Work up to 10 repetitions.

Partner Upper-Body Challenger

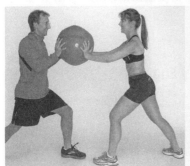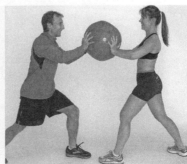

Face a partner and hold a weighted ball between you at chest level. Both of you will, in unison, push the ball toward each other. Each will take turns exerting more pressure forward while the other exerts less. Alternate pushing the ball back and forth. This is a fantastic movement for the core, arms, and overall upper-body strength.

Kneeling Balance Drill

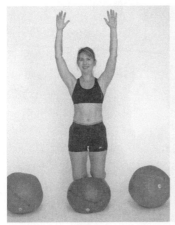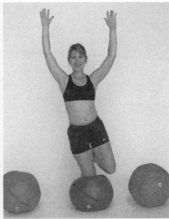

Softer weighted balls (not harder medicine or fitness balls) make fantastic balance and core challengers. Kneel on the ball while keeping both feet off the floor. Lift the arms over the head and hold for 20–30 seconds. If this is too easy, practice balancing on only one knee.

Partner Catch and Throw

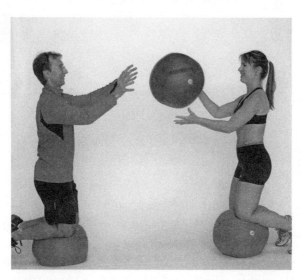

This drill requires the use of three fitness balls, two of them semi-soft to take pressure off the knees. Face your partner while you're each balancing on your knees on a soft weighted ball, with your feet resting on the floor. Toss the third ball back and forth while balancing. To make the drill more difficult, lift both feet off the floor and balance only on the knees while playing catch. Work up to 5–10 repetitions. Throwing a weighted ball back and forth with a partner builds strength and stamina. The additional element of balance turns the movement into a multidimensional drill.

Ball-Supported Plank

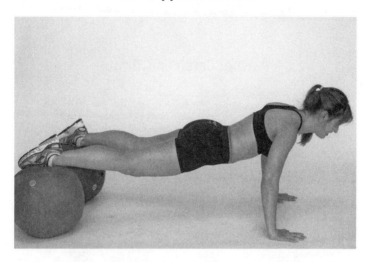

Practice a plank with the feet resting on one ball or each foot resting on a separate ball. Using one ball keeps the legs closer together, while using two moves them wider apart. Both variations challenge the core, arms, and back for a tremendous workout. Keep the back straight without slouching the shoulders. Try to time the plank, increasing the time to 30 seconds while maintaining good form. You can also work on push-ups in this position.

Ageless Agility

If you played hopscotch as a kid, you essentially used a type of agility ladder. This tool is fun because it allows movement in different directions and challenges our feet and brain with many patterns. We can run or jump at a steady pace in and out of the enclosed boxes, either forward, sideways, or backward. The agility ladder helps improve our speed, balance, coordination, and strength.

As you've probably guessed, an agility ladder isn't something to prop up against a wall to reach high places. They're made of durable, lightweight plastic or flexible fabric. This means that they're portable and versatile since they take up very little space and can be used on any flat surface, both indoors and outside. If you don't wish to buy an agility ladder, you can build your own, using any number of materials such as wood, tape, rope, or shoelaces. You can even draw one with chalk on the ground. The typical ladder is made up of 18-inch squares and is about 16 feet in length, but you can create any dimensions that appeal to you.

The number of movement drills we can perform with the agility ladder is unlimited, which brings the fun element into practice since we're able to express our creativity in making up motions that appeal to us. To improve agility, we can jump into the empty spaces between the rungs of the ladder and make our way to the end as fast as we can. These motions also help train our fast-twitch muscles and improve our reflexes. The ability to react quickly can be beneficial, and changing body position instantly is an attribute we can all use.

Combining linear and lateral movements helps the body-mind connection and improves physical mechanics, coordination, and balance. Continually practicing footwork drills assists in increasing our stamina and cardiovascular fitness. Agility-ladder exercises may include simple movements, such as lifting the knees high while running sideways, or more challenging skills, such as jumping in and out of a box with both feet simultaneously. Ladders can also provide an excellent, dynamic warm-up.

Diagonal Footwork

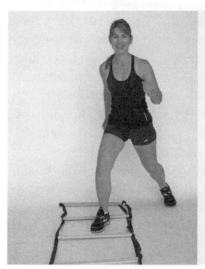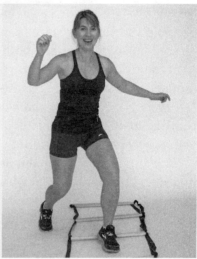

Start at one end of the ladder. Angle the body slightly diagonally and move into the first square with the right foot and follow with the left. Move out of the square on the opposite side of the ladder, leading with the right foot and following with the left. Continuing to work diagonally, move into the next square with the left foot followed by the right. Move out of the square on the opposite side of the ladder, leading with the left foot and following with the right. You should be traveling into a different square each time, gradually making your way down toward the end. Work on perfecting these patterns before increasing the speed and duration of the drill.

Sidestep Running

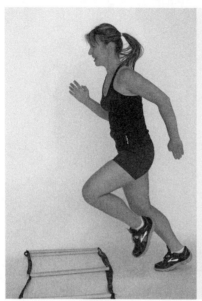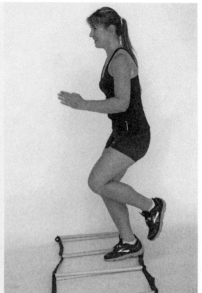

Face the long side of the ladder. Beginning on one end, run forward inside the ladder square with the right foot, followed by the left foot. Return to starting position by placing the right foot back followed by the left. Now move into the next square in the same way, making your way down the length of the ladder until reaching the end. Alternate the feet and travel back in the opposite direction. Focus on accuracy first before working up to increasing the speed.

Hopscotch Fun

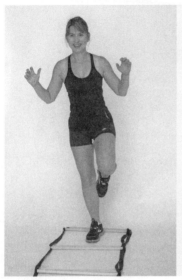 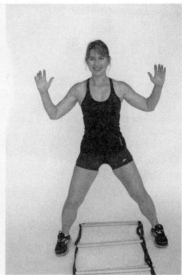

Pretend to play hopscotch by hopping into the ladder square with one foot and jumping out with both feet straddling the ladder. Alternate feet.

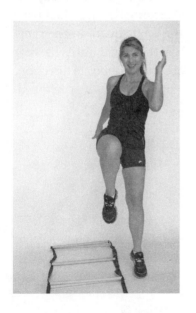

Knee-Ups

Begin by standing next to the ladder, placing your right foot inside the ladder square. As soon as the right foot touches the square, lift the right knee toward the ceiling, maintaining your balance while hopping slightly forward with the left foot. When lowering the right knee, place the right foot inside the next forward square. The motion will be similar to walking forward and raising the knee of the right leg, except you'll be using the ladder to gauge where to place the right foot. Only the knee inside the square will be raised, and the left foot will remain outside the ladder for the duration of this drill. When you reach the end of the ladder, turn around and work the opposite leg. Adding swinging motions with the arms to any ladder drill will help increase the heart rate and provide a greater challenge.

Traveling Ladder Push-Ups

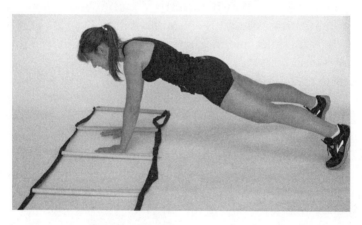

Place both hands inside a ladder square in push-up position. Begin to walk the hands into the next square, one at a time, while stepping with the feet in the same direction. Maintain a straight back. Lead with the left arm, then switch and lead with the right arm. Feel the arms, core, and back working. For a more challenging motion, do a push-up before walking the arms into the next square.

Smooth Rolling

Anyone who has experienced the pleasure of a massage understands its value in easing sore muscles and fostering relaxation. A foam roller—a cylindrical piece of hard-celled foam, available in various density levels—allows us to become our own personal, advanced masseuse. It has become a popular fitness tool during the past decade and is no longer just a staple of the physical-therapy community.

Foam rolling is sometimes called *myofascial release* because we work on the soft connective tissue located just below the skin, which is called *fascia.* It wraps and connects the muscles, bones, nerves, and blood vessels of our body. Along with our muscles, it makes up the myofascial system.

Through lack of use or improper movements, our fascia and the underlying muscle tissue can become "stuck" together. This can lead to adhesions, which restrict muscle movement, leading to pain, stiffness, and reduced flexibility. Even if we stretch regularly, sometimes muscle knots don't go away and lead to pain and stiffness.

The foam roller allows us the unlimited ability to self-massage with a small monetary investment in the tool itself. It lets us apply a solid, controlled load on the body, and this gentle application of pressure on sensitive muscles massages knots and helps the tissue relax. As the muscle we're rolling becomes soothed, blood flow and circulation are increased. Consistent, daily application over time can help break down soft tissue adhesions and scar tissue, helping to improve range of motion.[8] It can also work to decrease soft-tissue injuries.

Rolling helps us get more in touch with our body by allowing us to distinguish between levels of discomfort that may be related to potential injuries. We have direct control of how often we wish to roll, as well as the amount of pressure we decide to exert on a given area of muscle. It's a wonderful way to warm up before we exercise, allowing for a better workout. Using a roller to cool down afterward aids in recovery from strenuous movements. It's relaxing to foam roll the body after a hard day at work, and smoothing out those knots can help release tension built up in our connective tissue, making us feel less stressed. Rolling can also keep us more flexible, especially crucial if we're sitting all day.

While rolling may feel slightly uncomfortable to some people initially, if you persevere, it becomes easier and more enjoyable. Work up to rolling once per day for at least 5-10 minutes.

Foam-Roller Movements

Leg Roller

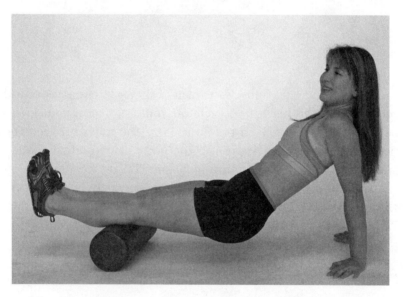

Rolling the legs, especially the calves, is important for increasing circulation and injury prevention. Calf muscles can become tight and painful, especially after standing on hard surfaces for long periods of time or wearing high-heeled shoes. Roll the calves gently, starting from the bottom and working up toward the back of the knee. Avoid going over any joints. Roll gently back down toward the feet.

Back Roller

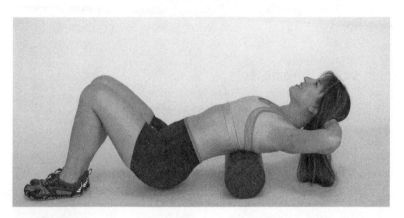

Rolling the back muscles can help increase circulation and break up hard-to-reach knots. Lie on your back with your knees bent and your feet flat on the floor. Place the roller between the floor and your waist. Slowly roll the body over the foam roller. Support your head with your hands, and control the pressure on the spine to avoid injury. Avoid rolling the neck. Notice where the muscles feel tight, and stop at these spots for several seconds. Remember to breathe slowly and deeply.

Gold-Star Equipment for Fun Movement

Investing in unique fitness equipment that challenges and excites us can be a motivating experience. Many of my clients have found success by placing a piece of compact fitness gear in each room of the house as a reminder to get in some movement. The following equipment is fun, interesting, engaging, and most of all, effective help with fitness goals. Seek it out online and enjoy it for years. A great idea is to temporarily trade gear with family and friends and then swap back every few weeks to keep things fresh.

Lifeline Power Wheel

The Lifeline Power Wheel was created by Jon Hinds, founder of the Monkey Bar Gym and vice president of LifelineUSA. It consists of a wheel with an axle through the center that provides fasteners allowing placement of the feet or hands.

The Power Wheel is designed to dynamically improve core strength, power, and balance; it also can work the upper body, hips, and gluteus. It's portable, easy to store, and allows us to make up unlimited motions to challenge these muscles. A strong core helps improve balance and power, decreasing the chance of injury because it helps stabilize the upper and lower body. It's a great piece of equipment for all fitness levels.

Power Wheel Knees to Chest

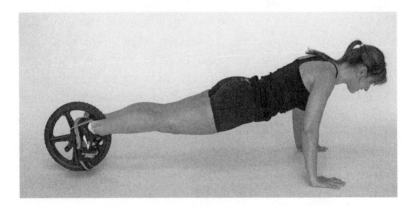

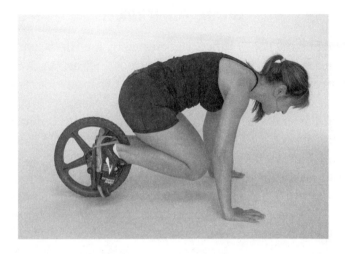

Start from a seated position and strap the Power Wheel to your feet securely. Gently turn over into push-up position and lift your body off the floor. Allow your arms to support your upper body while your feet remain strapped to the wheel on the floor. Keep your knees off the ground and focus on body alignment: Try to maintain a straight line from your head to your feet. Using your core and legs, roll the wheel forward by bringing your knees up toward your elbows, keeping the wheel on the floor. Feel the core, legs, and arms working. Extend back to starting position. Work up to 10 repetitions several times per day.

Slide Board

Slide boards have been used by speed skaters and hockey players for years and are gaining popularity today as more people start to find out about their benefits. During childhood, many of us loved to find ways to slide on any slippery surface. We loved gliding on ice, roller skating, and slipping around on Grandma's freshly waxed floor.

A slide board is a slick plastic mat that has blocks on each side, which are used as stoppers (bumpers) to push off. Cloth-like booties are placed over the shoes to allow smooth movement across the mat (socks can be used as well). Most slide boards have adjustable bumpers that can be set at various widths. The farther apart, the more force must be exerted to slide from one end to the other, and the greater the strengthening effect.

The hip is one of the most common sites for problems, and the majority of us aren't performing hip exercises that counter prolonged sitting. The hip is very similar to the shoulder in that they're both ball-and-socket joints, capable of moving in many directions. Many of us are simply not moving or strengthening our joints enough to counter a sedentary lifestyle.

Strong hips are important because they have to support the weight of our entire trunk and provide mobility for the entire body. This is where the slide board comes into play because it strengthens each aspect of the hips and hip stabilizers through closed-chain exercises, which means the foot is in contact with the floor. This type of movement enhances compression forces that stabilize the joints and help prevent injury. Sliding is one of the few thigh exercises that can be performed as a closed-chain movement, making it very beneficial.

Incorporating the slide board into our movement repertoire adds variety and is a great way to get our cardiovascular conditioning done, all while reducing the risk of hip injuries. Remember to start off very slow in the beginning. Then increase the duration as needed. You'll soon feel the benefits, and friends and family members will definitely want to try something that looks like fun—so prepare to share!

Side Sliding

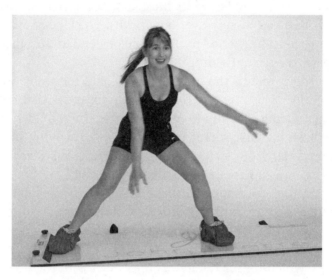

The board featured in these photos is made by Ultraslide. Sliding back and forth is a fun and challenging workout. Simply start at one end of the board and propel the leading leg toward the opposite side. It's okay if you don't make it all the way across during the first few tries. Keep working at it and your legs will build up the required strength with time. Enjoy the feeling of sliding from side to side.

Mountain Climber

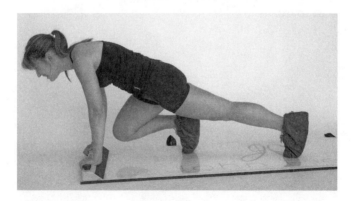

From a crouching position, firmly hold the slide board bumper while placing both feet on the board. Alternate moving one foot toward the bumper while moving the other foot back. Keep your back straight during the motions and feel the core and legs working.

Flexi-Bar

Flexi-Bar is a handheld oscillating device that vibrates when we exert muscular force. The vibration is what helps affect the deep muscles of the body while positively influencing muscular strength, joint mobility, and injury recovery. Using our own power to vibrate the bar means that we're in complete control of starting and stopping the motion. The body responds to the vibrational training by initiating both the voluntary and involuntary muscles, engaging a greater number of muscle fibers. This helps increase blood flow.

As the bar's vibrations pass through the body, they push and pull the muscles out of equilibrium. These contraction signals travel continuously to the brain by way of the nervous system. The signals challenge the muscles, forcing them to automatically contract in order to bring themselves back to a balanced position.

All major muscle groups can be worked, including the shoulders, abdominals, lower body, triceps, and biceps. Since strong core muscles are essential to spinal integrity, working this area is crucial to help avoid injuries. Training with the bar is also fun and unique. It can be used while standing or sitting, making it particularly useful for those in wheelchairs and beds.

The bar is lightweight (just over one pound) and is suitable for beginner fitness enthusiasts or dedicated athletes because it uses your own strength and technique to increase the progressive intensity of the workout.

Triceps Challenge

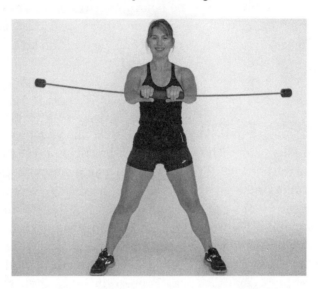

Hold the Flexi-Bar in front of the body, keeping the elbows slightly bent and the palms facing the floor. Gently push the bar back and forth, feeling the challenge in the triceps. Work up to 30 seconds several times per day.

Enjoy these fitness modalities and continue to experiment, play, and use your imagination and creativity to make up movements that feel fun, challenging, and engaging. Invite more motion into your day the way so many of my clients have—by placing your favorite fitness equipment in each room of your home as a helpful reminder to use them often. The more you come back to moving, the more your health will flourish.

CHAPTER 9

COUNTERING OUR SITTING LIFESTYLE

Do you ever stop to think about how much you sit during the day? Chances are great that you're sitting down right at this moment. How is it that many people complain of fatigue when all they do is sit all day? Shouldn't they feel more lively since they haven't been exerting much physical energy? It may seem that way, yet the opposite is true: We think we're conserving our energy but end up feeling exhausted when we get home after hardly moving at all.

Today, sitting in a slumped-over posture for countless hours has become a daily prison for millions of Americans and many others around the world. Our sedentary lifestyle is a recent cultural disaster. Fifty years ago, the majority of people didn't attend gyms, yet very few struggled to maintain a healthy weight. Today, technology has slowly leached hundreds of calories out of our day. For thousands of years, we worked for a living with sweat on our brow, using our arms and legs, engaging all of our muscles. Now, many of us earn an income by sitting all day while using only our fingers to type information into a computer. This lack of movement is guiding us toward obesity, stiffness, lethargy, and ultimately, illness.[1]

Many health experts recommend physical movement for 30 minutes during the day, but what about the other 23.5 hours? *What we do for the rest of the day is critically important. It may mean the difference between life and death.*

Our bodies adjust to what we do most often. If we sit all day, we become best adapted to sitting. The problem is that this makes us *less* proficient in running, jumping, and squatting. We should all be able to perform these movements with some skill, yet many of us cannot. The chair can't offer us motion because it's specifically designed to force us into immobility.

The solution to prolonged sitting is simply to stand up and stretch, bend, twist, reach, and walk around frequently. Gentle, leisurely motions stimulate the nervous system, which helps keep us alert and maintains blood flow to the brain. Just adding standing and sneaking a few motions into our sitting routine can increase circulation, muscle tone, and energy and burn extra calories. The cure for prolonged sitting is not more gym exercises but simply *not sitting* as much without much movement.

Strategies for Thriving in a Chair-bound Society

Take a look at the following suggestions for counteracting pro-longed sitting situations. Becoming more conscious about our posture and the time we spend on our seats will allow us to change our habits and increase our health as a result.

— **Try a different posture.** Changing or modifying our common sitting position helps improve our circulation and energy levels. We don't have to sit the conventional way, especially at home. We can be cross-legged or have our knees up, as shown in the following photos. Experiment with what feels best and try to shift positions at least several times every hour. Notice how your body feels in the different positions.

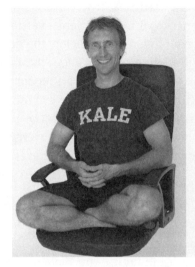 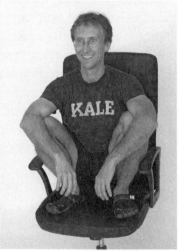

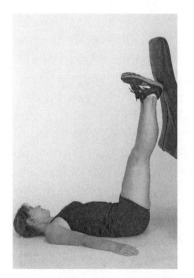

— **Lie down on the job.** It's a good idea to lie down for a few minutes to stretch if you're feeling fatigued and stiff during the day. Bring a yoga mat or towel to use as floor padding, and lie down while stretching the back and legs gently. Prop the feet up against a sturdy chair or wall if possible. Remember to breathe and relax completely for several minutes.

— **Get a headset or use a speaker.** Holding the phone between your ear and shoulder can create neck pain that radiates all the way down the arm. A hands-free device or a speaker can help keep the neck aligned. When talking on the phone, make it a habit to stand up and pace or walk around to improve circulation and burn additional calories.

— **Adjust the computer screen.** Staring at a screen for hours can lead to eyestrain and cause neck pain. To prevent eyestrain, position the center of the screen seven to ten inches below the horizontal line of vision and a little less than an arm's length away. Look away from the screen at least every 30 minutes and focus on an object about 20 feet away. Shifting focus and regular eye movements lessen the risk of eye irritation and headaches. Make sure your computer and desk lighting are adequate. Dark screens or small fonts can cause you to squint, frown, and strain your eyes.

— **Take the stairs.** Taking the stairs (if it's safe) for just five minutes a day, five days a week, can help us lose more than two pounds over the course of the year. A 150-pound person will burn an average of seven calories per minute walking up the stairs, compared to just one calorie per minute taking the elevator. Any additional walking we can fit into the day all adds up.

— **Consider the stand-up desk.** These are gaining popularity in many workplaces, and standing burns three times as many calories as sitting. There are also desks with integrated treadmills that allow walking at a slow but steady pace while you're working. If standing is an option, use wooden risers under an existing desk to elevate it or stack large books under your keyboard. If you're considering standing while typing, begin slowly and gradually increase the time to avoid sore legs. Make sure the surface you're on is soft enough to support standing for longer periods of time and that you wear comfortable shoes.

— **Remember to breathe.** Most of us have a tendency to hold our breath, especially when we're under stress or engaged in challenging mental work. This decrease in oxygen to the brain and muscles can make us feel lethargic and tired. Keep work spaces well ventilated, especially with fresh outside air if possible. Bring in small plants—living ones, not plastic—to decorate the desk or work area. Plants help deliver much-needed oxygen to indoor areas with poor air circulation and help us connect with nature in a small way, even when we're in front of a computer all day. Just glancing at some green leaves or a flower has the power to make us smile. Remember to take deep breaths several times per hour and try to stay conscious about excessively holding the breath.

— **Become aware of the body while sitting.** We frequently don't focus on our body position when we engage in strenuous mental tasks. Without checking in, back pain and other signs that we're out of alignment may go unnoticed. If you're not aware of your body signals or choose to ignore them because you're too busy, you become used to the discomfort and avoid doing anything about it. This may lead to problems in the long term. When you're mindful of how your body feels, you can make physical adjustments that will allow you to feel better. Make it a point to connect with how your body is feeling and check in often to see whether a quick walk or stretch is necessary to revive body and mind.

— **Massage for circulation.** Giving yourself frequent hand, finger, arm, leg, and foot massages is a healthy way to stimulate circulation. Massaging helps break up knots and reduces pain stemming from poor function. Touch helps release tension. Even the palms of the hands have a fair amount of muscle. One way to sneak hand and arm massage into the day is during driving stops. Whether waiting at a red light or in bumper-to-bumper traffic, you can use the extra minutes to gently squeeze and massage the forearms, wrists, palms, and fingers. If you're sitting at a desk for long periods of time, try to remove your shoes and massage your feet and toes.

— **Use a footstool.** Many people of shorter stature can't sit comfortably in conventional chairs, since they're designed to fit someone of a particular height. Ideally, it's best to have the heels flat on the floor, but many chairs simply don't allow this, causing only the toes to touch the floor. When this happens, the seat delivers constant pressure to the backs of the thighs, which can lead to pain and fatigue. Be sure your heels meet the ground firmly and use footstools, telephone books, or a sturdy box under your feet to help with the proper alignment.

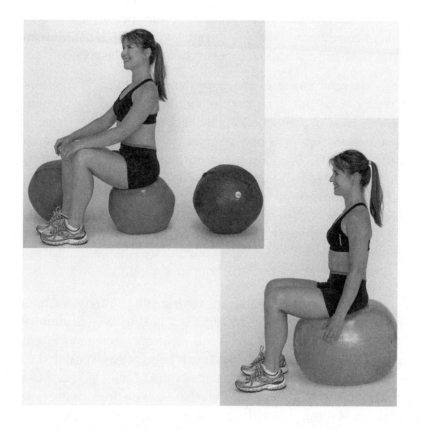

   — **Sit on a Swiss ball, medicine ball, or similar weighted ball.**
Sitting on a relatively unstable surface such as a Swiss ball requires
us to use our legs and encourages our torso and different muscles
to actively engage continually. This helps overcome some of the
circulation problems and muscle fatigue resulting from sedentary
work. The added benefit is an alert mind. Changing up the seat
periodically, such as switching to a medicine ball or other weighted
ball, encourages a greater range of movement and works different
muscle groups. Beginners can begin by sitting on a slightly deflated
ball, which requires less balance and effort, and then increase the
density of the ball with time, as balance is improved.

— **Stretch the arms.** When the muscles of the arms and wrists feel tired and stiff, take a few minutes to stretch them. Move the chair away from the desk while raising your arms in front of your body and open them at shoulder level. Stretch the chest and back as if you're trying to hug the back of the chair with your arms. Keep the palms facing the ceiling as if two cups of water are being balanced on them. Note how your upper body is feeling. Try to incorporate this stretch several times a day. We often have a tendency to slouch forward, and gently stretching back helps counter this habit.

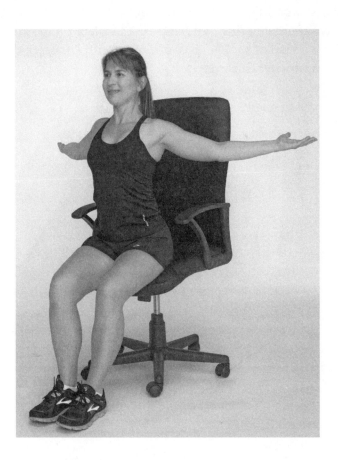

— **Strengthen the forearms.** This part of the body is often neglected in many fitness regimens and needs to be challenged regularly to maintain and improve arm strength. Grab a thick fitness band (as shown in the photo) and extend the arm in front of the body, keeping the elbow fairly straight; the knuckles will be facing the ceiling. Allow the band to hang down toward the floor. Begin to scrunch the band together while pulling it up and into the hand with a grabbing motion. Take time with the motion, pausing to squeeze the fitness band gently as it moves farther away from the floor and accumulates in your hand. Feel the forearm and wrist working. This motion should start to feel challenging quickly. Alternate arms. If a band isn't available, you can substitute a long scarf or similar piece of cloth. Gently massage the wrist and forearm after this exercise.

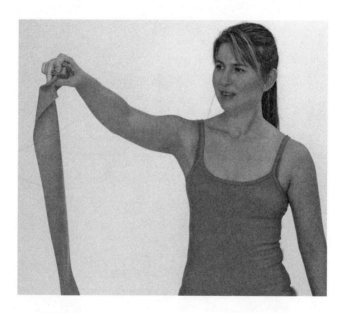

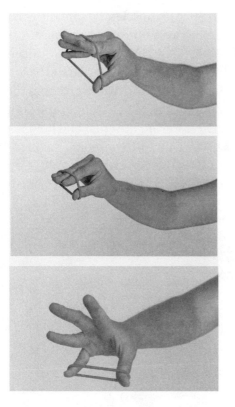

— **Strengthen the fingers.** We frequently take our fingers for granted and don't give them additional exercises that can be useful for keeping them strong and flexible. Common rubber bands or hair scrunchies make convenient and affordable finger strengtheners. Place the band around the fingers and touch all five fingertips together, forming a point. Draw the fingers apart against the resistance of the band like a reverse squeeze. Feel the effort the fingers are making. Try to work up to 10 repetitions with each hand. Variations include slipping the band around the thumb and one of the other four fingers, then drawing them apart against the resistance.

These exercises can easily be done while sitting at a desk, on the bus, on an airplane, or anytime you like. Most of us are far stronger gripping with the fingers than going in the opposite direction. Notice which fingers and hand are weaker, and then work them more. Hair bands come in various thicknesses and sizes, allowing us to keep challenging the fingers by choosing thicker bands as we progress.

— **Use the chair to strengthen core muscles.** Be sure the chair is sturdy, especially the armrests, to avoid breaking the furniture and causing injury. The chair should be stable to avoid any sudden rolling movements. This is a challenging motion that should be initiated slowly. Begin by sitting in the chair and firmly grabbing the solid armrests. Slowly lift the body out of the chair by using your arm strength. Try to lift up the knees toward the chest and hold the position as long as comfortable. Work up to 10 or more repetitions during the day. The first photo shows the beginner's basic position and the second is a more advanced version with the legs extended.

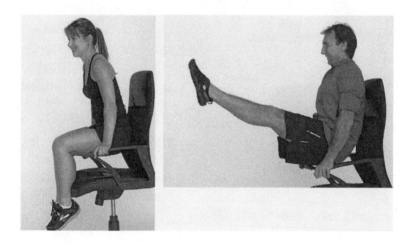

— **Remember the neck.** Don't forget about your neck if you're sitting for long periods of time. It can become stiff, especially if you hold the same flexed-forward position all day. Slowly turn the head from side to side, noting which side feels more flexible. Look up at the ceiling and down at the floor. While looking forward, gently bend the neck and try to reach the ear toward the shoulder. Hold each position for a few seconds or as long as it feels comfortable. Always stretch the neck very slowly and gently.

— **Squat.** The majority of us don't incorporate squatting into our daily activities and miss out on the benefits offered by this overlooked and underestimated motion. It's an effective posture that stretches the back musculature and opens the hip joints. It also stimulates the legs, core, back, and gluteus muscles.

Squatting can be performed with or without equipment, virtually anywhere and anytime. Many elderly seniors in Eastern cultures are able to perform deep squatting positions because of consistent practice and sitting close to the ground, without the use of chairs. We can all acquire this ability with practice, patience, and time, gaining health benefits as a result.

How to squat: Depending on your level of flexibility, you can initially practice with a rolled-up blanket, towel, or shirt under the heels. If you're new to squatting, it's a good idea to start with your back close to the wall for additional support in keeping upright.

Each of us squats in a unique way. The shape of our bones, hips, and thighs ultimately determines what's natural for us. Some of us have our feet parallel and knees closer together, while others squat with the legs apart and feet turned out. Find the position that feels best. Practice often, slowly increasing the time. One of the best ways to improve is to practice during television commercials, gradually working up to holding the position for the duration of the break.

Try squatting while wearing shoes or barefoot and feel the difference in flexibility. These photos shows a basic squat with a rolled shirt under the heels and a full squat.

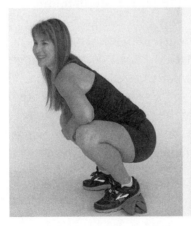 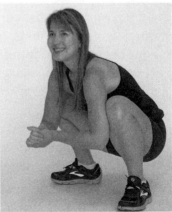

Unbinding Our Feet

Our foot is the first interaction between our body and the earth. We're all born without shoes because humans don't require footwear to stabilize our joints or keep our lower-leg tissues healthy. Numerous cultures have been living happily for thousands of years without $150 gym shoes.

Feet are vital for whole-body balance and contain thousands of sensory nerves that collect information on temperature, pressure, and environmental terrain. When we bind ourselves in ill-fitting shoes, it can feel as if a straitjacket has been forced upon us. Most footwear limits the natural motion of our joints during walking, leading to increased back pain. Since there's hardly a human movement that doesn't involve the feet, if we neglect to properly care for them, our balance is compromised and we become prone to falls and ankle sprains.

Wearing high-heeled shoes is a crippling experience for many women. Not only do the shoes frequently cause pain, but they may also lead to lifelong issues such as foot instability, bunions, back problems, and calluses.[2] The knee is negatively affected by wearing these unnatural contraptions and may be one of the reasons for the higher incidence of osteoarthritis in this joint in women compared to men.[3] Wearing high heels over many years may also compromise muscle efficiency during walking, leading to muscle pain and fatigue, while increasing the risk of strain injuries.[4]

Studies have found that cushioned shoes significantly impair our awareness of foot position compared to less structured shoes.[5] This is one of the reasons minimalist footwear is gaining momentum as people begin to gravitate instinctively to choices that allow them to feel the earth. The less shoe "support" we provide our feet, the greater their ability to evaluate the ground, allowing more communication between the foot and the environment. I encourage my clients to go barefoot at home whenever possible. They also enjoy wearing minimalist shoes like Vibram FiveFingers.

Sole-Saving Tips

- Walk barefoot at home. This allows your feet to move naturally and have some quality "air time," exposed to the environment. Keep your floors free from tripping hazards and objects that can injure the bottoms of your feet.

- If you live close to a sandy area, it's a great idea to walk barefoot on the sand (being careful to avoid stepping on sharp objects). If you're sitting at the beach, try to grip the sand with your toes as a pleasant and stimulating exercise.

- Take off your shoes while enjoying outside activities such as picnics or concerts. Every opportunity to remove your shoes should be enjoyed. Your feet will appreciate this and reward you with greater foot health.

- Sitting at work while wearing tight, uncomfortable shoes can sap your energy. Try slipping off the shoes whenever possible to allow air time and increased circulation. Massage the feet often by gently but firmly squeezing the heel and the rest of the foot. Give each toe a few seconds of attention by gently bending it back and forward, similar to stretching the fingers.

- Use essential oils on the soles of the feet for additional relaxation or stimulation. A small drop of lavender oil in a foot cream helps us unwind before going to sleep. A drop of grapefruit oil around the ankles in the morning can help energize us for the day. Avoid applying creams directly to the feet before wearing shoes as they can cause the foot to become slippery and unstable inside the shoe.

- Commit to buying comfortable shoes without high heels to save your feet from long-term damage. Foot health is more important than making a fashion statement (especially a painful one).

- If wearing high-heeled shoes is necessary for a particular occasion, wear flats while driving and walking to the event. Keep a bag containing the flat shoes handy so that you can slip into them when the occasion is over.

- Enjoying a foot-bath is relaxing and refreshing. Try filling a small tub with water, add a few drops of an essential oil, and soak your feet. They'll love you for this.

- Let's vote with our dollars for shoes that are cruelty-free (vegan) and made with fair labor practices.

Challenge yourself daily by incorporating the tips outlined in this chapter, and continue to gradually add more movement into your day. By becoming more conscious of the time you spend sitting and following the simple motion suggestions in this book, you'll start to see positive changes in your energy levels, emotions, and overall health. Every bit of movement makes a difference. Your body will thank you for your efforts with increased physical performance and vitality.

Part IV

THE PILLAR OF COMPASSION

CHAPTER 10

THE UNIVERSAL ANTIDOTES

Throughout this book, I've focused on sharing nutritional, brain-building, and fitness-enhancing modalities. The final pillar of health is perhaps the most important because it holds the key elements that support and reinforce the rest.

We can eat the most healthful diet and exercise consistently, but if we allow the negative energies of anger, jealousy, hatred, and greed to destroy our spirit, then we—and our planet—have little chance of thriving. This is why the pillar of compassion is so critical.

Compassion opens the heart and encompasses many benevolent qualities: love, caring, kindness, warmth, sensitivity, tolerance, tenderness, and mercy. These are the priceless antidotes that defuse violence, fear, anger, and hatred, transforming us and the world for the better. Cultivating and focusing our energies on positive attributes is desperately important, today more than ever.

Love is at the heart of who we really are. Love is what we're all looking to manifest more of. When we fan the flames of kindness, generosity, and goodwill within us and our children, we thrive as a society. Our very happiness and the survival of our planet depends on our ability to cultivate loving and unselfish qualities.

In this chapter, I'll discuss some of the challenges that take people away from their naturally compassionate selves and share stories that express the miraculous healing power of this critical pillar of health.

Infectious Thoughts

Although the number of pollutants found in our food, air, and water is astronomical, the dangers they pose pale in comparison to the most destructive toxins found in our society today: hatred, anger, jealousy, and fear. These harmful emotions are often caused by our systematic focus on negative thoughts. Continually concentrating on and surrounding ourselves with detrimental energies prompts them to spill over into our being and eventually morph into our actions. Over time, they begin to dominate and define the very reality we experience. While we eat only several times per day, we generate *thousands* of thoughts daily, and it's these countless ponderings and deliberations that guide our destiny toward vibrancy or despair.

If we visualize ourselves as sponges that absorb and integrate the beliefs of our culture, being surrounded by pessimistic attitudes allows these harmful influences to seep into our consciousness, much like grime saturating a sponge. If the mind is continually showered by an acid rain of negativity, once happy and energetic people may turn into lethargic and depressed individuals.

We're often oblivious to the omnipresent influence society has on our mental patterns. A typical day, for many of us, often begins with an intrusion on our thoughts and feelings by the expertly choreographed words and graphic images of today's media. To escape the negativity we hear on the news, we turn on the radio with the hope of listening to uplifting music—yet we're often confronted with violent lyrics and alarming innuendo. The continual bombardment of the fertile mind with grim news, shocking gossip, sensationalized stories, manipulative commercials, and negative music continues throughout the day.

These trespassers violate our naturally harmonious nature, throw us off balance, and make us feel as if we're living in the twilight zone. Like a deflated boxer who's been beaten down from too many fights in the ring, we begin to feel mentally defeated and spiritually drained.

Pessimistic thinking can also be compared to a ruthless virus that infiltrates our being to cause mayhem. We may begin to have trouble falling asleep at night from excess fear and worry. In turn, the lack of physical and mental rest can ignite and exacerbate pain and sap our energy levels, stopping us from exercising, eating well, and even smiling. Since negative thoughts are highly opportunistic in nature, the weaker their host, the faster they proliferate.

When we believe that we can't effect change for the better, a persistent feeling of annoyance and discord begins to exude from us and overflows to everyone we come across. Just as small children unwittingly infect playmates with the flu through a cough or sneeze, we often become unconscious carriers of cynicism, jealousy, and despair. We may contaminate others with our harsh, bitter words and rude behavior—becoming impatient and snappy with the grocery clerk, yelling and shaking our fists at fellow drivers, and glaring angrily at kids who act rambunctious in restaurants. This inner tension and friction is passed on to friends, family, co-workers, and society as a whole. They, in turn, pass it back to us and everyone else around them, much like spreading a contagious cold or flu.

Thankfully, there is help. Just as we can decrease the chances of catching a cold or the flu by washing our hands frequently and encouraging others to cover their mouth and nose when they sneeze, we can similarly help prevent the spread of harmful emotional viruses and defuse them with the helpful methods you'll read about next.

Uplifting the Atmosphere

Creating a more joyful environment in our home can be a powerful tool to change our thoughts for the better. If our dwelling is filled with clutter, dust, and reminders of sadness, the effect on our psyche will be detrimental. However, if we surround ourselves with pictures, decorations, and other items that bring us delight, we're reinforcing the positive. Every time we look around and smile, our brain will release feel-good chemicals, making us feel better. The more we smile and exude happiness, the more we and others are affected in a positive way. Since most of us have direct control of the items we bring into our home, making a change for the better is a doable and often pleasant activity.

One of the most successful environment-enhancing tools that I introduce to new clients is a collage. Chances are great that you made a collage during art class in school, but if you didn't, know that it's made by securing photos, pictures, quotes, or drawings to a sheet of paper or a piece of cardboard.

I have my clients cut out pictures from magazines of their favorite surroundings, such as a forest or a beach, and add photos of the activities they enjoy, such as bike riding, running on the sand, swimming in the ocean, or making sand castles with their kids. They display these "happy posters" anywhere they like at home. I encourage them to write down affirmations next to the scenes, such as: *I am attaining this vision easily and effortlessly,* or *This is my destiny.*

Many of my clients make several collages and place them in different rooms. Some make a small one to carry in their purse or wallet. This allows them to take something positive with them anywhere they travel and helps uplift their spirit when they need a quick visual boost.

Essential oils (discussed in detail in Chapter 6) are also powerful mood enhancers to incorporate in your home. Simply spraying the air with your favorite oils, diluted with water, can help increase your happiness. In addition, the oils improve indoor air quality and make rooms smell pleasantly fresh. Carrying a tissue with a drop of your favorite oil in your pocket or purse allows you to smell the tissue at any time, almost anywhere, for instant refreshment or relaxation.

The continual bombardment of doom-and-gloom news can contribute to a negative atmosphere. Unplugging from the depressing information can help improve our moods. Taking care in choosing which shows deserve our time is important. Picking programs that further encourage us to make our home beautiful, organized, and inviting is wonderful inspiration.

Inviting more joy into our work space is also important since we tend to spend a great deal of time at the office. Being surrounded by healthy plants, happy photos, and other uplifting items such as inspirational quotes and positive affirmations can help us feel happier on the job.

Listening to pleasant music is a quick way to uplift the atmosphere for the better. Recordings of nature, such as birds, dolphins, or ocean waves, are pleasant and add a positive mood to our space. Incorporating pleasant wind chimes both outdoors and indoors brings a delightful element of magical sound.

Enhancing our surroundings helps to tremendously uplift the spirit—but perhaps the greatest remedies we possess all originate from compassion.

The Power of Compassion

Teaching and lecturing over the years has allowed me to witness the unlimited capacity of love and compassion to heal and transform countless lives. Perhaps one of the most powerful narratives I share with my audiences is the story of Lisa.

As a small child, Lisa suffered unimaginable abuse when her parents indoctrinated her into a cult. The years of trauma and horror inflicted on her body and psyche left a deep scar in her sense of self. Understandably, Lisa had doubts about people's intentions and continually feared being harmed by others.

If children are bathed in negativity, hate, and violence, these detrimental toxins begin to imprint themselves on the psyche. When they're continually told they're worthless and ugly, they start to believe it. Since Lisa was blamed for the pain others inflicted on her, she internalized the belief that she deserved misery and deplorable neglect. She was programmed to view herself as inherently bad. These damaging, persistent thoughts defined her reality and morphed into self-destruction. Even though Lisa spent three long decades looking for help and emotional support with psychiatrists, psychologists, and other health professionals, she continued to brutally injure herself, and it seemed no relief was in sight.

When I first met Lisa and heard her stories of terror, it was difficult to stop the tears from coming to my eyes. Perpetuating cruel acts on an innocent child can be called nothing less than evil. It was a miracle that she was still alive and functioning.

Lisa didn't believe that unconditional love existed because her childhood environment was saturated with fear, pain, confusion, and darkness. She couldn't fathom that kindness and compassion existed in other people. Because her body and mind were drenched in destruction and negativity for years, her psyche critically needed an immersion in positivity, light, peace, safety, and kindness. Little did I know that extending compassion would prove to be the astoundingly powerful catalyst to the healing she'd been desperately seeking.

Lisa's remarkable breakthroughs began almost immediately. When she mentioned during our first session that she couldn't afford to see me again because of her limited budget, I assured her that I would continue to help her free of charge. This stunned her and left her momentarily speechless. She had never received anything without being asked for something in return. No one had ever offered true caring and compassion. When Lisa told me that she could not afford to shop at the health-food store for the ingredients I recommended, I let her know that I would buy the groceries for her. These simple gestures of kindness were so shocking that she asked me if this was a trick, because her childhood taught her that people only took whatever they wanted from her in ways that caused grief and suffering.

Knowing how critical a supportive home environment is for attaining peace of mind and contentment, I helped Lisa transform her house into a positive, inviting, and safe sanctuary by decorating it with pictures of uplifting angels and happy smiley faces. We placed positive, encouraging, and heartwarming affirmations in every room, and even her car. Lisa became surrounded by optimistic words and cheerful drawings of virtuous and kind beings. This had an uplifting effect and made her smile often. She also began to write down affirmations every day, listened to uplifting music, and watched inspiring DVDs. These positive influences helped her feel better, and her positive momentum continued to build.

Miraculously, after only two sessions, Lisa stopped physically abusing herself after years and years of unproductive therapy. This astonished her. She never thought that she could stop injuring herself, especially in such a short time. While I'm not a doctor or a psychologist, I assert that many people reading this could have helped Lisa by simply sharing and offering true unconditional love, empathy, and caring.

After those first two sessions, I continued to work with Lisa on the phone, through e-mail, and in person so that she was continually surrounded by positive feedback and encouragement. For the first time in her life, Lisa felt cared for. Love and kindness were the antidotes she had been desperately needing. Once she experienced these miraculous healing attributes, she stopped hurting herself and started to exude serenity and peace.

Think Good Thoughts, Do Good Deeds

Clients and friends are used to hearing me say, "Think good thoughts and do good deeds." This has been my mantra for many years and sums up my philosophy in a nutshell. The power of uplifting thoughts and the beauty of good deeds create a *synergy of immense positive power*. The more energy we invest in thinking about kindness and compassion, the more inclined we become to put those ideas into real actions that have profoundly favorable effects. Negative thoughts leave a blazing trail of destruction, not only in the body, but also in our vulnerable mind.

Becoming more loving and compassionate starts with our thoughts. Thinking is the active energy that paves the way for the physical manifestation we call reality. If we hold on to our good intentions without turning them into actions, who will benefit?

I once visited a yoga studio where many of the students and instructors wore white robes and walked around in a serene, meditative state. They dwelled on good thoughts and exuded tranquility and peace while on their yoga mats. As I went to use the restroom in this establishment, I was taken aback by the complete disarray. It looked as if a hurricane had hit indoors. Paper towels and garbage lay all over the floor, and water was everywhere. I took the time to clean up the restroom and wiped everything down, never thinking that this was not my responsibility.

Our good thoughts must expand into good deeds to affect our surroundings for the better. *We're all connected, and extending a good action to others is the same as extending it to ourselves.* As I finished cleaning and closed the door behind me, I jokingly said to myself, *That, my friends, is yoga.* You see, the meaning of *yoga* is unity, spirituality, and discipline. These are qualities that one does not just practice while others are watching or when we're at class. The people in the studio who were well aware of the trashed state of the restroom did not take any action to make it better. While they may have felt peace inside, they did not act to spread that tranquility into their immediate environment. Their harmonious thoughts were not demonstrated in the world.

When we become peace and act upon our sense of unity, *we live it everywhere we are,* not just on our lunch break or during a meditation class. Thinking good thoughts is a step in the right direction, but *doing good deeds initiates the physical manifestation of that thought,* changing reality for the better. The actions solidify everything into the life we experience.

Softening Hearts

I originally started teaching fitness boot camps more than ten years ago to empower young women in high school and college. My goal was to motivate them to be physically stronger and more emotionally resilient. While many traditional boot camps focused on aggressive tactics and used derogatory words to motivate their attendees by "breaking them down," I always filled the class with positive words and ideas. I specifically designed it to be a support- ive and uplifting experience, where everyone worked at her own individual pace and encouraged the others.

I vividly recall a new girl coming into the class wearing a hooded sweatshirt, headphones, and black nail polish. Initially, her attitude was negative, and she didn't interact or communicate with anyone. As the months passed, she slowly began to transform. Not only did her attitude change, so did her physical appearance.

One day during class, I inquired about what had happened, since she now resembled Snow White. I'll never forget what she said: "You just softened me." It made me happy and proud that she was able to change her life just by being in an environment filled with positive young women. Everyone was there to help each other. I only had two rules: First, that everyone respect her body's limitations and move at her own speed. This helped foster respect and consideration toward each person's individual fitness levels. Second, I highly encouraged these young women to support and uplift one another. Rallying around others not only strengthens and motivates the people we're inspiring, it also influences us for the better.

I never turned any girl away, even if they couldn't pay for the class, because my goal was to instill positive energy into the lives of these young women. The money didn't matter to me because enhancing their lives was priceless. Regardless of how negative someone may seem, as long as they're continually "bathed" in a positive atmosphere and surrounded by a supportive network overflowing with care, love, and compassion, they can transform themselves for the better.

Turn a Frown Upside Down

Seeing the goodness in others begins with compassion. Life will always present us with situations that test our ability to choose between negative or positive behaviors. If our thoughts are focused on *seeing the goodness in others,* our actions will manifest those beliefs.

More than 30 years ago, I worked at a health-food store. One customer was an unfriendly woman who acquired a negative reputation for being rude and argumentative. When she came in, everyone seemed to disappear to avoid her tantrums. I was a fairly new employee and only heard about her from the other employees. Even though I didn't have any personal interactions with her, I still viewed her with the same kindness and compassion as everyone I met. My only goal was to help others, and I considered the store to be a place of healing and positivity, where people could find supportive products for body, mind, and spirit and meet with other health-minded individuals.

One day, the woman came in during my shift. I did my best to help her find the items she was looking for, and when she was ready to pay for the groceries, I offered to ring her up. She began asking me questions about supplements, but seemed annoyed when I offered her useful answers. It quickly became apparent that she was ready to get into a verbal confrontation.

We kept some expensive sample gifts under the counter for customers who spent more than $100, and I asked her if she'd like some, even though her bill didn't amount to very much. She gazed at me with bewilderment.

When I handed her a gift, her expression changed from confusion to utter disbelief, while I continued to give her more presents. My goal was to show her that she was cared for and accepted, regardless of her poor attitude. I wanted her to experience the positive energy and joy the store offered, and I genuinely wanted to help her.

She looked at me silently for what seemed like eternity, and then finally said, "You know, no one has ever done anything like that for me before." Her demeanor changed completely. She smiled, perhaps for the first time in a long while. A simple gesture of kindness and generosity can melt the fear and anger around a wounded heart, breaking it out of a self-imposed hate prison.

Expanding positive thoughts to ourselves and everyone around us starts with a desire to be more loving and compassionate. The more we focus on looking for ways to act with kindness, the more we can help change the world for the better. Our circle of goodness will then continue to grow, embracing everyone we meet with compassion.

All Beings Need a Compassionate Hand

Recently, I was leaving someone's house to get to the airport. I was trying to hurry so that I wouldn't miss my shuttle and, consequently, my plane. Suddenly, time seemed to stand still as I noticed some ants on the kitchen floor as I walked toward the door. One ant seemed to be trying to free herself from what appeared to be a sticky substance. (Interestingly, almost all "worker" ants are female.)

Completely forgetting my shuttle and where I needed to be, I gently picked up this sticky ant with a piece of paper and put a bit of water in my palm, gently placing her in the droplet. As she floated, I shook my hand to vibrate the water, giving her a Jacuzzi bath, washing off the stickiness. I touched a paper towel to the water in my palm and it sucked the moisture up, leaving the ant standing there, all clean. I placed her back on the ground, and she went about her business without further restrictions. I didn't miss my shuttle after all, and I didn't miss my plane—but most important of all, I didn't miss out on the priceless opportunity to help a precious living being in need.

All expressions of life are sacred. This little ant's life is just as important as the majestic whales or an elephant. We shouldn't discriminate against other beings based on size or appearance any more than we should judge people on their looks. Many individuals enjoy fuzzy, furry animals but can't tolerate other humans. This is species discrimination and also applies to those who like humans but not animals. Why is it okay to love poodles but not spiders? Dogs but not cows? Sheep but not pigs? At the end of the day, we either serve love or we serve hate. The choice is up to us.

Mother Teresa is reported to have said that the smallest deed done is far greater than the greatest intention. We can think many grand thoughts about helping the world, but if we do nothing, what have we changed for the better? Small good deeds done, when accumulated over time, can accomplish more than grand acts pondered but never begun.

Even knowing this, it's still easy to become overwhelmed and feel immobilized by the sheer amount of need that exists in the world. That's one of the reasons I started the 5 Minute Activism page on my website (www.johnpierre.com). I provide links to other websites that have prewritten letters asking for change or voicing concern about worthy causes, such as the compassionate treatment of animals, the preservation of our environment, and humanitarian issues. It takes just a few minutes to sign a letter you feel strongly about and click "Send." In that short amount of time, you can make a positive contribution to the world!

Spending even a few minutes on worthy causes does more good than putting all of our thoughts into majestic dreams that are never acted upon. Helping others empowers us, too, and can make us feel wonderful.

In the closing chapter, I'll discuss ways we can cultivate more compassion to help ourselves and others thrive in fantastic ways.

CHAPTER 11

CULTIVATING COMPASSION

We sometimes hear people describe others as seeing life through rose-colored glasses, meaning that they're choosing to see the more positive side of things. What would it be like if we looked at the world through the lens of compassion?

Seeking opportunities to act with care for others and seeing ourselves in a new light can change us all for the better. In this chapter, I'll share some of the ways we can cultivate more compassion and gain the immense rewards of opening each other's hearts.

Lowering Our Drawbridge

In the past, many castles and fortresses were purposely surrounded by deep lagoons and ditches around their outside walls to discourage invaders. When castle residents chose to permit visitors entry, a drawbridge was lowered to form a solid walkway that allowed passage inside. When the drawbridge was lifted again, it became an impenetrable wall that kept intruders away.

If we visualize our body as a castle that houses our mind and spirit, we can begin to use the drawbridge analogy as a metaphor for allowing people into our emotional space. When we decide to keep our drawbridge up, closed, and sealed in interactions with others, they meet an unyielding wall that impedes full connection and understanding.

We often put up walls because of fear. Many people feel uneasy about sharing their true thoughts and perceived weaknesses with others because it opens them up to potential rejection and ridicule. Wearing a mask to impress others seems to be the only solution to stay safe from judgment. The problem with disguising our true self is that we become liked for being someone we aren't, rather than who we are inside. In many ways, it's better to be disliked for being our true self rather than loved and admired for who we're pretending to be. The exhausting effort of maintaining a facade eventually takes its toll, and we start to feel resentful toward the very individuals we tried so hard to impress.

Sadly, many people continually keep their drawbridges up, thinking they'll be safer emotionally, never allowing others to get to know them on a deeper level. This robs everyone of their inherently good qualities just because they fear not fitting into society's current fads, ideas, and whims. Having the courage to extend our bridge to others opens our heart to a fuller emotional connection, which can be a satisfying and healing experience on both sides. There are numerous ways we can lower our drawbridges, and many of them don't cost a single penny.

Smiling Attracts Joyfulness

Perhaps the most underestimated and underutilized "bridge" we all possess is our ability to smile. Human babies instinctively know the power of a smile and use it often to transfix their parents, the adults making goofy faces and using funny, cartoon-like voices. These interactions reward everyone with joyous laughter.

Receiving a warm smile can change our mood from sad to happy. Likewise, when we extend a sympathetic smile of understanding to someone who is nervous, we offer them comfort and acknowledge their concerns. Smiling puts everyone at ease. Laughter and harmless joking are a great way to connect. They help us establish a sense of security. When we feel safe, we can let down our guard—the drawbridge can be lowered—and we can communicate fully.

Too many people are wearing permanent frowns, and many don't experience a smile for days or even months. That's tragic, because it's a strong indication of internal unhappiness. We all instinctively yearn for joy and contentment and are drawn toward those who express these qualities. Keeping the "smile bridge" open may lead to heartfelt interactions and help pave the way to enjoyment and fulfillment.

We're led to believe that we need to have specific reasons to smile, but this is not the case. We can smile simply for the joy of it, without any obvious cause. Just the physical expression releases feel-good chemicals in the brain, which communicate with every part of our body, making us feel better. If we try to smile more often, we'll notice the positive effect it has on the people we meet as well as on our own well-being.

Smiling is a powerful antidote to negativity and a strong bridge to well-being. When we're genuinely happy and compassionate, hate, rage, jealousy, and fear have a difficult time infecting us. This upbeat expression becomes our shield, much like antioxidants keep harmful rogue elements immobilized in our body. And when we smile at others, we offer them the antidote to negative emotions by lifting them up out of bad moods. It's a win-win for everyone.

Offering kind gestures such as genuinely inquiring about another person's day or just saying "Hello," helps us connect and communicate. It feels wonderful to extend warmhearted care and sincere concern. The considerate acknowledgment of offering a "Thank you" when someone goes out of their way for us makes everyone feel appreciated. We often feel the honest intent of others. If we send thoughts of well-being to everyone we meet, our actions will start to mirror our good wishes.

Extending Compassion

When I first began working in the geriatrics field, I learned a valuable lesson about the power of compassion. Since I was new to conducting senior seminars and work groups, I arrived early to set up the classroom with elaborate props, connect the VCR (not DVD player) to the television properly, and make sure everything was prepared. I began to notice that many seniors arrived very early, sometimes an hour in advance, simply because they were excited about the lecture and wanted to connect and communicate with someone.

The more experience I acquired in geriatrics, the more I began to understand the debilitating loneliness our senior population faces in retirement facilities, nursing homes, and adult-care centers. These establishments are often a microcosm of society. Some seniors in wheelchairs purposely isolate themselves because they feel different. Others may separate themselves because they had a stroke and can't speak coherently, which makes them feel embarrassed. The more walls people build that disallow expression and communication, the lonelier they feel, regardless of how many others happen to be in the same room. With every exhalation, they seem to be dying emotionally from the feelings of isolation and separation.

I purposely began arriving earlier, sometimes by more than an hour, even when my setup didn't require much time, just to talk with those already anxiously awaiting some company and connection. People's transformations are often remarkable when they're given tender, caring attention and understanding. *A kind acknowledgment and a compassionate ear are often more powerful than any advice.* Just the expression of real feelings is often sufficient to help people feel happier. Seniors who initially looked lethargic and depressed transformed into energetic and joyous individuals. They were ecstatic to connect with someone and eager to share their memories, present trials, and future hopes.

A kind, platonic touch, when appropriate, can serve as another compassionate bridge to help people connect with one other. "Failure to thrive" is a condition that occurs in human newborns and baby animals when they're not touched and caressed. They lose the ability to ward off infections effectively and can even die. Similarly, many adults in our culture are failing to thrive because a compassionate touch and considerate affection aren't offered to them.

I learned just how crucial it is to make a small physical connection with seniors by simply talking with them, listening to their challenges, holding their hands, or putting a hand on their shoulder. Many hadn't been touched for years. A simple, small gesture of loving touch made all the difference in the world to them.

When I think of extending compassion, I often remember an elderly blind woman who always came to my lectures at her retirement home. She arrived early and talked to me about her life, and we often chatted until class began. She sat in her wheelchair at the back of the room and listened intently to my lectures, often nodding and smiling at the information I was presenting. When the class ended, I'd come over and speak with her again, to continue our connection. She always thanked me for taking the time to communicate with her, and even though she couldn't see me, she could hear the genuine caring in my words. She told me that she enjoyed coming to my seminars early just to hear my voice.

I often wondered how much interaction she had during the day. Was I one of the only people who reached out to her? We often presume too much about others' lives, thinking our positive impact isn't really needed or wanted, but that is often not the case. Extending compassion through positive interactions not only affects them tremendously, but overflows in miraculous ways.

Another memory that continues to have a profound effect on me is of a homeless man in my local community. As a young adult, I often took fruit, juices, and peanut butter and jelly sandwiches in quantities to distribute to the homeless people in needy neighborhoods. On a certain day, when I completely ran out of the food and juices I brought to give out, I noticed a homeless man who looked thirsty. Luckily, there was a store nearby, and I quickly ran in to buy a juice drink. When I handed it to him, I expected him to open up the bottle and gulp down the liquid immediately. To my surprise, he walked over to another homeless man and offered to share. This man clearly had no home or material possessions, and was in desperate need of hydration. Yet the small extension of compassion he received from me, he was willing to pass along to another person, sacrificing his own needs.

We all have the power to affect one another either negatively or positively. Extending compassion can invite meaningful interactions that are beneficial to everyone. Opening our hearts by smiling and reaching out with care pave a way toward fulfilling connections, greater understanding, and the sharing of hopes and dreams.

Raising the Moral Bar

As a culture, we've been undergoing a steady metamorphosis of declining ethics and morals. Hardly anyone bats an eye anymore when television programs, cartoons, and most recently, reality shows, glorify violence, abuse, narcissism, greed, and mean-spirited behavior. In fact, many of these disturbing presentations become instant hits, acting as the fixative that cements us to the couch for hours. We become desensitized to the hostility we see around us because we're submerged further and further in a spiritually deprived society. The more we witness and experience the deterioration of dignity, respect, honesty, and integrity, the easier our compliance and acceptance becomes. Embracing mediocrity and lowering our internal codes of conduct seem to be the only options that allow us to fit in.

Lowering our principles is often encouraged not just by the media, but also by those who seek to justify their own behavior. Others may stand to benefit from our moral submissions. Bosses may encourage us to look the other way when a work error places their bonuses in jeopardy. An acquaintance could coax us into having a piece of cake when we're struggling to lose weight. Daily scenarios test our virtues and shift our internal standards. The lower our inner-value set point becomes, the more easily we succumb to harmful behaviors that may hurt others and erode our self-respect. Many of us are not living up to our own expectations, and we can certainly do better as a society.

Those who have made the most positive impact have always lived by a high code. These are the people history often applauds for having honor, loyalty, and selflessness. Mother Teresa and Gandhi are two such individuals, and there are countless others we can look to for inspiration.

Keeping a "moral mentor" in our mind's eye is helpful when we're faced with an ethical dillema. "What would [fill in the blank with your personal moral hero] do in this situation?" is a question people use to help with such predicaments. Striving to raise our personal ethical bar can work wonders, both for us and for those who may be inspired by our actions. If we cease to compromise, and continue trying to do better, life will mirror our integrity.

As a young child, I often ran to the corner store for snacks. On one occasion, after buying some items, I stuffed the change into my pocket and headed home. After walking for about three blocks, I dug the money out of my pocket and counted it. I discovered that the clerk had given me more change than I was due. Without thinking twice, I turned around and went back, giving the shocked cashier the extra money. Sadly, people aren't used to others being honest, especially when it comes to money.

What does it say about our world when truthfulness is viewed with suspicion and distrust? In the decades I've been placing orders with businesses, when I've found an error in my favor, I've always brought it up. The employees of many companies encouraged me to just keep the extra products or not pay the difference. Many were simply baffled that someone would offer to give them the money they were owed, since they'd never know about it if I didn't bring it to their attention.

When I contacted establishments that overpaid me for my work, I was often told, "What are you complaining about? Just keep the money." Although most people would have been delighted, it made me sad that the employees didn't want to go through the trouble of correcting the error, even though it was to their company's financial benefit.

Do we need to raise the moral bar in our lives? Our society's influence is eroding our ethics and self-esteem by repeatedly lowering morality. When a stream flows over a boulder, the seemingly harmless water, *over time,* has the potential to erode and split the rock in half. Just as powerfully, low cultural standards continue to flood us—and our innocent children—with lower and lower values.

Raising our principles begins with asking ourselves more questions and holding ourselves accountable for our actions. Becoming conscious about what the most honorable action would be in a given situation and taking responsibility boosts our self-esteem and builds internal strength. Raising our bar of ethics and morals helps everyone in society.

Questions to Raise the Bar

- How can I increase my expectations for my diet?
- What are the obstacles that keep me from increasing my health and energy levels?
- How can I raise my standards in my interactions with others?
- How can I be a role model for good morals and values?
- What values am I teaching my children or the young people in my life?
- What principles do I stand for?
- Am I respectful of the ethical beliefs of others?
- How can I do better as an individual and help our society?

Getting into the habit of questioning our ethics and continually striving to lift them sets an example and builds our confidence. If everyone operated with the highest morals, what would our trusting and honest world look like? By continuing to raise our standards, we can live a more valiant life and begin creating that world today.

Zooming in on the Positive

Imagine attending a celebration where everyone is having a wonderful time socializing, smiling, and laughing. A camera crew walks in to film the scene for a nightly news segment, but focus their lens on only a limited area. The spot they capture happens to include a couple angrily arguing in the corner for the duration of the shoot. When the footage is broadcast later, it seems that this party wasn't fun at all because of the discord the couple showed. This gives viewers a false impression and the portrayal of the party is inaccurate and incomplete.

We all possess a camera in our mind that can either enhance or downplay the significance of different situations. We can focus on what's positive or what's negative. We can see people as good or bad, right or wrong. That does not mean we should turn a blind eye and not notice any negativity. We just don't want to focus on the unpleasantness *continually.*

How often do you use your internal lens to emphasize mistakes, resentment, and grievances? In school, miscalculations were pointed out; we were taught to look for errors to avoid making them. Many of us became accustomed to searching for what's wrong instead of focusing our mind on what's right.

We're often rewarded for noticing problems at work, too, and we start to get stuck in that pattern, always looking for and picking up on the negative. This makes people good at their jobs in finding errors, but can easily spill over into other areas of life, such as raising kids and marriage.

Similar to our immune system, which is on guard for things being out of place, paramedics, police officers, and firefighters all offer us protection, playing a critical role in society. In working with military and law-enforcement personnel for decades, I've noted a common denominator: Because of job influence and training, these people's internal cameras look for and focus on what's wrong outside of work—expired license plates, a missing taillight, speeding motorists, and erratic behavior. The problems arise when they turn their critical and error-seeking eye on their family members, friends, and spouse.

Focusing the internal camera lens consistently on the negative breeds suspicious thoughts that cast shadows on loved ones. It encourages doubt, uncertainty, and insecurity. When the kids come home later than usual, we wonder if they're doing drugs. When our spouse leaves to take a call in another room, we wonder if they're deceiving us. We radiate criticism and suspicion to everyone around us.

The answer is to start to consciously train the brain to search for positive situations. Focus on reclaiming and investing attention in what's right. Looking for the good is a significant catalyst to positive outcomes. The more we scan the world for good things, the more we find. The more we zoom in on what's encouraging, the more favorable the outcome.

Words Can Hurt or Heal

"Sticks and stones may break your bones, but words can tear your heart apart" is a saying I often use to emphasize the powerful effect words exert on our physical and mental health. They can invoke peace and tranquility or division and disharmony.

Our brain responds to the impressions made by the words we see, hear, and speak. Words create graphic pictures in our mind, and these vivid snapshots directly influence our feelings, moods, and actions. When we sense a particular feeling or belief, the brain sends out hormones and chemicals, which then change the physiological processes and reactions of our body. If we watch a scary movie, our heart begins to pound, we often gasp at some of the scenes, our body becomes tense, adrenaline starts racing, and our breathing quickens. Yet all we're looking at is a screen. How are these reactions possible when we know that we and the actors are quite safe and it's all just make-believe? The answer is this: The brain does not know the difference between what we see and what we pretend to engage in. The mind just responds. This is why words are so powerful. *Words create images in our mind that evoke the same physiological responses as experiencing the visualized action.*

A brief verbal exchange has the power to make us laugh or cry. The spark from a fiery tongue can burn down relationships and communities. When people experience uncontrolled rage, they sometimes fire off words similar to bullets released from a gun. Once launched and fired, those negative sentiments can't be taken back and end up inflicting lasting damage.

Are we acting as if we're living in a reality TV show, looking for more drama, using abusive words and making sarcastic comments about ourselves and others? It's common for people to use negative phrases without thinking about it because everyone else is saying the same thing: "I hate that," or "My job is killing me," and the phrase recently popular with teenagers to express that something is good, "That's sick!"

We might be surprised by how many times a day we hear, say, or think negative remarks. It seems like more people voice their complaints about others than their compliments. Kind words don't cost money, yet many of us act as though speaking them out loud will deplete some imaginary bank account. Caring, considerate, friendly, and well-meaning comments are needed today more than ever before. They have the power to elevate us, to make us feel joyous, loving, and enthusiastic. Words possess the power to heal.

It feels good to say pleasant things—just the act of voicing positive phrases can put us in a good mood, *changing us physiologically.* Statements of concern for others' well-being create a greater state of harmony within us. It's a gift to everyone and attracts more of the same back to us. Most people are rarely listened to, much less understood or validated. Even the smallest kind word extended to another can bring out powerful gratitude.

Do you use phrases like *Thank you* often? If you make that one statement a daily habit, you'll start to gain incredible rewards in being a happier person. When we hear and say, "Thank you," we acknowledge that we're grateful. It's not important if we're thankful for something small, like someone holding the elevator for us, or large, like receiving a special gift. How many times have we opened the door for someone only to see them walk right by without saying anything, or let someone go ahead of us in traffic but never received a friendly wave in return?

Of course, the idea is to do good without getting anything back, but it always feels nice to be acknowledged for going out of our way. Hearing a warm "Thank you" accomplishes this and makes everyone feel better.

Let's focus on being more conscious of the words we're speaking daily. Begin to listen intently. Try not to judge or retaliate when you hear something negative. Simply be a neutral witness, without reaction. Take pleasure in offering pleasant words to people and appreciate listening to amicable conversations. Brighten someone's day by saying something kind. The warm feelings from a compliment or a comment that shows we care can keep both us and the recipient smiling for hours.

Choosing Words Wisely

We're all worthy of kind words. The perfect time to be kind with those we love is now, so they know exactly how we feel. We often take them for granted, feeling that they'll always be around, but that's often not the case.

Surprisingly, people we judge as negative or unfriendly are often the ones who can use kindness the most. When I spoke with seniors in retirement homes, I often posed the following scenario to the audience: How would they feel, as they went back to their room for the evening, if another senior stepped into the elevator and began arguing with them? Would they say something short and sharp back? If everyone went to their respective rooms in foul and angry moods, what would happen if they learned that the person who started the argument passed away in their sleep the same evening? How would they feel if they knew that the last words the angered person heard on this planet were their negative retorts? All of the seniors agreed that they'd feel terrible and many had tears in their eyes at the mere thought.

What if we turned the situation around and said to the individual who was snappy with us, "It sounds like you're having a tough day. How can I help? What can I do to be of assistance to you?" How would we feel if we found out the person had passed away later that night? Sad, but at least we would have known that their last conversation was with someone caring, who reached out with compassion and love. The seniors always wholeheartedly agreed that this would make the biggest difference in the world to them. Speaking with kindness and cultivating an empathetic viewpoint makes a meaningful difference.

Sometimes, *how* we say something becomes more important than what we say. Paying attention to our tone, especially when we're trying to convey something positive, can be vital. If we have a sarcastic pitch, our favorable messages can take on a very different meaning from what we intend.

Our facial expressions and physical gestures also speak loudly, even though we may not utter a sound. Humans unconsiously look at these signals. If we're speaking to someone while reading, watching television, or blasting music through our headphones, they automatically get the impression that they're not as important as our entertainment. Fully listening to the person speaking helps that individual feel important and valued, regardless of whether we agree or disagree with their statements.

Cooling potentially damaging words starts with substituting more uplifting phrases. Take a look at some common sayings below and see if better words can be used.

Calming Word Eruptions

Common Volcanic Phrases	Calming and Uplifting Phrases
I hate this!	*I'm not thrilled about this.*
I'm depressed.	*My mood is momentarily lackluster.*
I failed!	*I'm in the process of learning.*
He/she is nasty!	*He/she is unique.*
I'm okay.	*I'm perfect.*
I'm dumb.	*I'm discovering my brilliance.*
I'm so angry!	*I'm temporarily annoyed.*
It didn't go as planned.	*Things may turn out even better than planned.*
I'm overwhelmed.	*It's nice to feel needed, and I'll do my best.*
I can't stand this!	*I'm not too keen on this.*

The Mess of Superficial Success

It's often said what matters most in life can't be bought with money. Yet we've been collectively convinced by marketing schemes to worship external wealth at the expense of connecting with our true selves and our loved ones in meaningful ways. Constant overstimulation by media, cell phones, and portable computers has kept us from tuning in to what's going on inside of us and what's truly important. In the quest to accomplish goals and become accepted and admired, we've lost touch with what's really fulfilling. We're being systematically hypnotized and lured into buying unnecessary stuff, and the results are predictable: immense debt, mountains of clutter, and emotionally bankrupt lives.

Almost every aspect of modern existence has become a commodity. Success is now largely defined by how many objects we can acumulate and how many zeros are at the end of our bank balance. In many ways, excessive possessions begin to act as domineering overlords, enslaving us with the constant worry of losing our money and fancy stuff. The more we have, the more we wonder if others like us for our toys or who we truly are inside. The more we accumulate, the more we must keep tabs on everything. When we hire others to help us keep track, we have to audit *them* to make sure they did the job properly.

This unrestrained focus on material distractions leaves us with less time to ponder and cultivate meaningful internal attributes or share moments with loved ones. Many of the teenagers I work with have the most current technological toys, but they freely admit that they'd trade them all for some quality time with their parents, who are too busy working to share a meal or watch their soccer games. Many children are given toys (bribes) to ease the guilty consciences of adults who don't want to make the extra effort or take the time to connect.

Today's monetary wealth is so unevenly distributed that we begin to assume that whoever has the most expensive stuff must be the happiest. We start believing that buying what others have will also make us feel better. But we're often disappointed when the new gadgets lose their sparkle.

Material success tempts us with a seductive illusion, trying to convince us that the sacrifices we make for new things are worthwhile and will alleviate our depression and despair. At first they provide an emotional rush, very similar to the high experienced by consuming processed sugar. However, a short time later, we come crashing down. We continue to work more so that we can accumulate greater heaps of money to buy additional objects that we think will bring us happiness. But we still feel unhappy—sometimes even more so, because the illusion that toys will bring us long-term happiness has been shattered. The more time we spend working and striving, the less time we have to stop and reflect on the important intimate relationships in our life, especially the vital relationship with ourself.

Hoarding money is similar to stockpiling food in locked depositories while people starve outside the doors. What good is it accomplishing if people aren't using it for necessities? The word *currency* reminds me of *current,* which describes the flow of water or electricity. Money should be fluid: some comes in, some goes out. Yet many continue to accumulate stagnant pools without allowing the wealth to circulate.

How many bank accounts sit overflowing but inactive, while others suffer around the clock from lack of water, food, and shelter—because of sealed-shut hearts and wallets? Even small bits of monetary help can be remarkable.

Modern society has done a magnificent job of diverting human attention from qualities that truly matter, such as integrity, honesty, and empathy, while magnifying the illusion that happiness can be found in greed, narcissism, and apathy. The truth is that continually searching outside of ourselves only provides temporary stimulation, but never *permanent satisfaction.* The answer is to move away from the limiting belief that we need excessive possesions to be happy. Serenity can be found within, not in material trinkets. Financial wealth opens the door to numerous opportunities to help others. In this way, it has the potential to change lives for the better.

The ancient pharaohs' tombs overflowing with vast riches all confirm that material bounties remain on earth after we pass on. When we take our final breath, our legacy is the enduring influence our words and actions had on others.

Last-Minute Wishes

Profound philosophers and sages of the past continue to serve as today's moral pillars. Through wise words and cautionary tales, they teach us that being kind and compassionate is the foundation of a spiritually happy and fulfilling existence. Their lessons stand the test of time because they're based on principles that are righteous and honorable.

Each of us has the potential to become that thought-provoking philosopher and the insightful teacher we greatly admire. Our words, both written and spoken, can have an everlasting influence. We can right the wrongs we see by taking positive actions every day. When we uphold our moral principles and help ourselves and others, we all move toward a better future. It's when we turn away from goodness that we run into disaster.

Working in the geriatrics field for so long has taught me that as people enter their final chapter in life, they often feel sorrow and disappointment for allowing the negative emotions of hate, anger, and jealousy to dominate many of their days. They're remorseful about the broken relationships they never mended and feel sorry for shouting bitter words that poisoned the hopes and dreams of others. They regret "stuffing money under the mattress" and not sharing it with their loved ones in times of hardship. They grieve over the petty grudges that resulted in years of eerily silent phones. If only they could just turn back the clock and do it all over . . .

While we can't rewind the time that's already passed, we can still deeply affect the days, weeks, months, and years we have before us. When we take care of ourselves by eating well and respect our body's needs for joyous movement, we help ensure that our health is vibrant and strong. When we support our cognitive abilities, we ensure that we maintain the ability to think clearly and intelligibly. When we listen to our compassionate inner voice and act upon its guidance, we conduct ourselves with consideration and reverence for all life.

As you begin to embrace and act upon the principles outlined in this book, the fear of last-minute regrets will begin to melt away. Anxiety will be replaced by renewed peace of mind and tranquility. Feeling exuberant physically, mentally, and emotionally will uplift you and encourage others to improve as well. Imagine the beauty of modeling your dynamic health and ethical choices to the world as you inspire your family members, friends, and everyone you meet. With a solid foundation of wellness, you'll pass on your eternal, brilliant heritage filled with love, gratitude, joy, and peace. Your lasting legacy. Your pillars of health.

AFTERWORD

Who creates our future? We all do. Together, we're generating a *shared* experience here on earth. Everything we think and believe eventually transforms into the actions that affect all living beings and our planet. We're all participating in this magnificent journey called life, and with renewed clarity, improved health, and greater compassion, we can create a more beautiful and joyous experience for everyone.

If we view ourselves as unique pillars that make up the structure of life on earth, the healthier we become, the greater our capacity to contribute positively to the world. When we're physically and mentally balanced, we acquire the energy we need to cultivate strong family bonds and solid community ties. This is why it's critical to build our health foundations.

It is my sincere wish that this book has motivated you to improve your dietary standards and has renewed your commitment to move your body more in fun and joyous ways. I hope that you feel inspired to expand your thinking and take care of your cognitive function. Your increased health and vitality will serve as your bedrock for increased well-being. With the numerous tools you now possess, I trust that you'll be moved to cultivate, develop, and spread the compassion you feel in your heart with others.

Your contribution as a strong pillar will help uplift, strengthen, and guide our collective power. As a result, our ability to do good will become magnified exponentially for the betterment of our planet.

RESOURCES

Books

The 4-Ingredient Vegan, by Maribeth Abrams and Anne Dinshah

21-Day Weight Loss Kickstart, by Neal D. Barnard, M.D.

The 30-Day Vegan Challenge, by Colleen Patrick-Goudreau

The 80/10/10 Diet, by Dr. Douglas N. Graham

Becoming Raw, by Brenda Davis, R.D., and Vesanto Melina, M.S., R.D., with Rynn Berry

Becoming Vegan, by Brenda Davis, R.D., and Vesanto Melina, M.S., R.D.

Breaking the Food Seduction, by Neal D. Barnard M.D.

The China Study, by T. Collin Campbell, Ph.D., and Thomas M. Campbell, M.D.

Compassion: The Ultimate Ethic, by Victoria Moran

The Complete Idiot's Guide to Plant-Based Nutrition, by Julieanna Hever, M.S., R.D., C.P.T.

Defeating Diabetes, by Brenda Davis, R.D., and Tom Barnard , M.D.

Disease-Proof Your Child, by Joel Fuhrman, M.D.

Eat and Run, by Scott Jurek

Eat Vegan on $4 a Day, by Ellen Jaffe Jones

The Engine 2 Diet, by Rip Esselstyn

Farm Sanctuary, by Gene Bauer

Finding Ultra, by Rich Roll

Foods for the Gods, by Rynn Berry

Forks Over Knives, by Del Sroufe, with Isa Chandra Moskowitz

The Happy Herbivore, by Lindsay S. Nixon

Health Can Be Harmless, by H. Jay Dinshah

Here's Harmlessness, by H. Jay Dinshah

The Lean, by Kathy Freston

The Love-Powered Diet, by Victoria Moran

Mad Cowboy, by Howard F. Lyman

Main Street Vegan, by Victoria Moran

The McDougall Plan, by John A. McDougall, M.D., and Mary A. McDougall

McDougall's Medicine, by John A. McDougall, M.D.

The Most Noble Diet, by George Eisman, R.D.

My Beef with Meat, by Rip Esselstyn

Out of the Jungle, by H. Jay Dinshah

Peace Pilgrim, by Peace Pilgrim

The Pleasure Trap, by Douglas J. Lisle, Ph.D., and Alan Goldhamer, D.C.

Power Foods for the Brain, by Neal D. Barnard, M.D.

Prevent and Reverse Heart Disease, by Caldwell B. Esselstyn, Jr., M.D.

Skinny Bastard, by Rory Freedman and Kim Barnouin

Skinny Bitch, by Rory Freedman and Kim Barnouin

Super Immunity, by Joel Fuhrman, M.D.

Thrive, by Brendan Brazier

Thrive Fitness, by Brendan Brazier

Uncooking with Jameth and Kim, by Jameth Sheridan, N.D., and Kim Sheridan, N.D.

Unprocessed, by Chef AJ, with Glen Merzer

Vegan Bodybuilding & Fitness, by Robert Cheeke

The Vegan Diet as Chronic Disease Prevention, by Kerrie K. Saunders, Ph.D.

Vegan for Life, by Jack Norris, R.D., and Virginia Messina, M.P.H., R.D.

The Veggie Queen, by Jill Nussinow, M.S., R.D.

Whole, by T. Collin Campbell, Ph.D., with Howard Jacobson, Ph.D.

The World Peace Diet, by Will Tuttle, Ph.D.

DVDs

Calorie Density, by Jeff Novick M.S., R.D.

Earthlings, by Shaun Monson

Eating, by Mike Anderson

Fasting, by Michael Klaper, M.D.

Forks Over Knives

In the Kitchen with John Pierre and Friends, by John Pierre

Lighten Up, featuring Jeff Novick M.S., R.D.

Sense and Nonsense in Nutrition, by Michael Klaper, M.D.

Unity, by Shaun Monson

The Unprocessed 30 Day Challenge, by John Pierre and Chef AJ

Vegan Weight Loss, by John Pierre

When Bachelor Meets Homemaker, by John Pierre and Kerrie K. Saunders, Ph.D.

Websites

www.johnpierre.com – John Pierre: articles, recipes, and links

www.compassionatecook.com – Colleen Patrick-Goudreau: plant-based information, podcasts, and more

earthlings.com – Earthlings DVD

www.eatunprocessed.com – Chef AJ: whole-food recipes and information

doctorklaper.com/index.html – Dr. Michael Klaper: plant based-information and videos

www.drfuhrman.com – Dr. Joel Fuhrman: plant-based articles and information

www.drmcdougall.com – Dr. John McDougall: health and nutrition information

www.forksoverknives.com – Forks Over Knives: health and nutrition information

www.healthforce.com – Dr. Jameth Sheridan: health and nutrition information, podcasts

www.healthpromoting.com – TrueNorth Health Center

www.healthychick.com – Dr. Kim Sheridan: fitness, body-care products, and more

jeffnovick.com/RD/Home.html – Jeff Novick, M.S., R.D.: information on health-related topics

www.kathyfreston.com – Kathy Freston: nutritional information and more

www.madcowboy.com – Howard Lyman: educational information on plant-based diet

mainstreetvegan.net – Victoria Moran: nutritional information and more

www.numitea.com – Numi tea: organic tea information

www.nutritionfacts.org – Dr. Michael Greger, M.D.: nutritional information, videos, and more

www.PlantBasedDietitian.com – Julieanna Hever M.S., R.D., C.P.T.: plant-based dietitian

www.pcrm.org – Physicians Committee for Responsible Medicine: information on health, nutrition, and ethical treatment of animals

www.ravediet.com – Mike Anderson: numerous nutritional resources and links

www.tcolincampbell.org – T. Collin Campbell, Ph.D.: numerous health resources and links

www.skinnybitch.net – Rory Freedman: nutrition information and more

www.sproutman.com – Superb resource for everything related to sprouting

unitythemovement.com – Unity film information

www.veganbodybuilding.com – Robert Cheeke: vegan bodybuilding

www.warriorforce.com – Dr. Jameth Sheridan: health nutrition information, podcasts

Companies

Blendtec – quality blenders; available at www.johnpierre.com: click Shop, Blendtec

Boku – superfoods, tea, plant-based protein powder; available at www.johnpierre.com: click Shop, Boku

Clearly Filtered – quality water filters, www.clearlyfiltered.com

Cutriwellness – quality supplements, essential oils, vegan cosmetics, www.cutriwellness.com

Dynamax – quality weighted balls, www.medicineballs.com

The Fanciful Fox – quality vegan soap and candle company, www.fancifulfox.com

Flexi-Bar – Information on Flexi-Bar and more, flexi-bar.com/us/en/home

Floracopeia – quality essential oils; available at www.johnpierre.com: Click Shop, Floracopeia

Happy Tiffin – stainless-steel containers for food storage; available at www.johnpierre.com: click Shop, Happy Tiffin

HealthForce Nutritionals – quality green powders, protein powders, and a wide variety of nutritional supplements; available at www.johnpierre.com: click Shop, HealthForce

Herb Pharm – quality herbal products, www.herb-pharm.com

Journey Bar – plant-based food bars, www.journeybar.com (use coupon code: johnpierre)

LifelineUSA – quality fitness products; available at www.johnpierre.com: click Shop, Lifeline

Now Foods – quality supplements, foods, essential oils, teas, and much more; many Now products are available at www.cutriwellness.com

Numi Tea – organic high-quality tea varieties, www.numitea.com

NuTru – quality vegan supplements, available at www.cutriwellness.com

Organic Food Bar – plant-based food bars, www.organicfoodbar.com

PurVen Corporation – quality air purifiers, www.purven.com

Power Systems – quality fitness products; available at www.johnpierre.com: click Shop, Power Systems

So Delicious – vegan cultured coconut milk, coconut milk, and much more, sodeliciousdairyfree.com

Solute ions – electrolytes, trace mineral drops; available at www.johnpierre.com; click Shop, Solute ions

Sunwarrior – plant-based protein powders, available at www.cutriwellness.com

Tribest – quality food dehydrators, juicers, and personal blenders; available at www.johnpierre.com: click Shop, then choose Tribest Dehydrator, Juice Extractor, or Personal Blender

Ugi – weighted fitness balls; available at www.johnpierre.com: click Shop, Ugifit

Ultraslide – quality slide boards and more, www.ultraslide.com

Vega – quality protein powders and nutritional support, myvega.com

Young Living Oils – quality essential oils available at www.cutriwellness.com

ENDNOTES

Chapter 1

1. "Latest Statistics on America's Overweight Population." PCRM: Physicians Committee for Responsible Medicine. http://www.pcrm.org/health/medNews/latest-statistics-on-americas-overweight (accessed October 12, 2012).

2. Greger, Michael, "Are Artificial Colors Bad for You?" NutritionFacts.org, http://nutritionfacts.org/video/are-artificial-colors-bad-for-you/ (accessed October 12, 2012); Greger, Michael, "Fast Food Tested for Carcinogens," NutritionFacts.org, http://nutritionfacts.org/video/fast-food-tested-for-carcinogens/ (accessed October 12, 2012).

3. "Some Foods Have Drug-Like Effects on the Brain." PCRM: Physicians Committee for Responsible Medicine. http://www.pcrm.org/search/?cid=2460 (accessed October 12, 2012).

4. Barnard, Neal D. "Big Food About to Lose Its Biggest Defense: Food Really Is Addictive." PCRM: Physicians Committee for Responsible Medicine. http://www.pcrm.org/search/?cid=2111 (accessed October 12, 2012).

5. Lisle, Douglas J. and Goldhamer, Alan, *The Pleasure Trap,* Summertown, TN: Healthy Living Publications, 2003; Le Merrer, Julie, Becker, Jerome A. J., Befort, Katia, and Kieffer, Brigitte L., "Reward Processing by the Opioid System in the Brain," *Physiological Reviews,* http://physrev.physiology.org/content/89/4/1379.full (accessed March 21, 2013).

6. Le Merrer, Julie; Becker, Jerome A. J.; Befort, Katia; and Kieffer, Brigitte L., "Reward Processing by the Opioid System in the Brain," *Physiological Reviews,* http://physrev.physiology.org/content/89/4/1379.full (accessed March 21, 2013).

7. Layton, Lyndsey. "David Kessler: Fat, Salt and Sugar Alter Brain Chemistry, Make Us Eat Junk Food." *Washington Post.* http://www.washingtonpost.com/wp-dyn/content/article/2009/04/26/AR2009042602711.html (accessed October 12, 2012).

8. Lisle, Douglas J. and Goldhamer, Alan, *The Pleasure Trap,* Summertown, TN: Healthy Living Publications, 2003

9. "How Fiber Helps Protect Against Cancer," PCRM: Physicians Committee for Responsible Medicine, http://www.pcrm.org/search/?cid=3605 (accessed May 26, 2013); "Colon Cancer: Prevention and Survival," PCRM: Physicians Committee for Responsible Medicine, http://www.pcrm.org/search/?cid=3569 (accessed May 26, 2013)

10. "Constipation." National Digestive Diseases Information Clearinghouse. http://digestive.niddk.nih.gov/ddiseases/pubs/constipation/ (accessed October 12, 2012).

11. Barnard, Neal D. "Diet and Diabetes: Recipes for Success." PCRM: Physicians Committee for Responsible Medicine. http://www.pcrm.org/search/?cid=129 (accessed October 12, 2012).

12. Lakhan, Shaheen E. and Vieira, Karen F. "Nutritional therapies for mental disorders." *Nutrition Journal* (January 21, 2008). http://www.nutritionj.com/content/7/1/2 (accessed September 3, 2012).

13. "Whole Grains Improve Insulin Sensitivity," PCRM: Physicians Committe for Responsible Medicine, http://www.pcrm.org/search/?cid=771 (accessed May 26, 2013); "Hypoglycemia and Diet," PCRM: Physicians Committe for Responsible Medicine, http://www.pcrm.org/search/?cid=155 (accessed May 26,2013).

14. Barnard, Neal D., "Breaking the Food Seduction," PCRM: Physicians Committee for Responsible Medicine, http://www.pcrm.org/search/?cid=1290 (accessed October 12, 2012).

15. Lisle, Douglas J. and Goldhamer, Alan, *The Pleasure Trap,* Summertown, TN: Healthy Living Publications, 2003.

16. "Moose." Wikipedia. http://en.wikipedia.org/wiki/Moose (accessed October 12, 2012).

17. McDougall, John A. *The Starch Solution.* New York: Rodale, 2012.

18. McDougall, John. "Diet-Induced Precocious Puberty." The McDougall Newsletter (December 1997). http://drmcdougall.com/newsletter/nov_dec97.html (accessed October 11, 2012).

19. "When Friends Ask: Why Don't You Drink Milk?" The McDougall Newsletter (March 2007), http://www.drmcdougall.com/misc/2007nl/mar/070300.pdf (accessed September 19, 2012); "Milk and Prostate Cancer: The Evidence Mounts," PCRM: Physicians Committee for Responsible Medicine. http://www.pcrm.org/search/?cid=156 (accessed October 12, 2012); Chen JC, Shao ZM, Sheikh MS, Hussain A, Leroith D, Roberts CT, and Fontana JA (1994), "Insulin-like growth factor-binding protein enhancement of insulin-like growth factor-i (IGF-I)-mediated DNA synthesis and IGF-I binding in a human breast carcinoma cell line," *Journal of Cell Physiology,* 158: 69–78, http://www.ncbi.nlm.nih.gov/pubmed/ (accessed May 26, 2013).

20. Duggan C, Wang CY, Neuhouser ML, Xiao L, Smith AW, Reding KW, Baumgartner RN, Baumgartner KB, Bernstein L, Ballard-Barbash R, McTiernan A, "Associations of insulin-like growth factor and insulin-like growth factor binding protein-3 with mortality in women with breast cancer," *International Journal of Cancer,* 2012, National Center for Biotechnology Information. http://www.ncbi.nlm.nih.gov/pubmed/22847383 (accessed October 21, 2012).

21. Ngamphaiboon J, Chatchatee P, Thongkaew T. "Cow's milk allergy in Thai children." *Asian Pacific Journal of Allergy and Immunology.* 2008. National Center for Biotechnology Information. N.p., n.d. http://www.ncbi.nlm.nih.gov/pubmed/19317338 (accessed October 12, 2012).

22. Campbell, T. Colin, and Campbell, Thomas M. *The China Study: The Most Comprehensive Study of Nutrition Ever Conducted and the Startling Implications for Diet, Weight Loss and Long-Term Health.* Dallas, TX: BenBella Books, 2005.

23. "Health Concerns about Dairy Products." PCRM: Physicians Committe for Responsible Medicine. http://www.pcrm.org/health/diets/vegdiets/health-concerns-about-dairy-products (accessed May 26, 2013).

24. Sonneville KR, Gordon CM, Kocher MS, Pierce LM, Ramappa A, Field AE, "Vitamin D, Calcium, and Dairy Intakes and Stress Fractures Among Female Adolescents," *Arch Pediatr Adolesc Med,* published ahead of print March 5, 2012; "Health Concerns about Dairy Products," PCRM: Physicians Committee for Responsible Medicine, http://www.pcrm.org/search/?cid=252 (accessed October 12, 2012).

25. "Preventing and Reversing Osteoporosis," PCRM: Physicians Committe for Responsible Medicine, http://www.pcrm.org/search/?cid=161 (accessed May 26, 2013); "New PCRM Study Shatters Milk Myth: Children's Bone Health Tied to Exercise, Not Dairy," PCRM: Physicians Committe for Responsible Medicine. http://www.pcrm.org/search/?cid=1202 (accessed May 26, 2013).

Chapter 2

1. Fuhrman, Joel, *Super Immunity: The Essential Nutrition Guide for Boosting Your Body's Defenses to Live Longer, Stronger, and Disease Free,* New York: HarperOne, 2011; Bergner, Paul, *The Healing Power of Minerals, Special Nutrients, and Trace Elements.* Rocklin, CA: Prima Publications, 1997.

2. Brazier, Brendan, *Thrive: The Vegan Nutrition Guide to Optimal Performance in Sports and Life.* Philadelphia, PA: Da Capo/Lifelong, 2008; Ornish, Dean, *The Spectrum,* New York: Random House, 2007.

3. "How Can I Get Enough Protein? The Protein Myth," PCRM: Physicians Committee for Responsible Medicine, http://www.pcrm.org/search/?cid=251 (accessed October 21, 2012); "Plant Foods Provide Nutritional Building Blocks to Optimum Health," Dr. McDougall's Health and Medical Center, http://www.drmcdougall.com/free_2e.html (accessed May 26, 2013).

4. McDougall, John. "Five Major Poisons Inherently Found in Animal Foods." The McDougall Newsletter. http://drmcdougall.com/misc/2010nl/jan/poison.htm (accessed October 12, 2012).

5. Greger, Michael. "Anti-Inflammatory Effects of Purple Potatoes." NutritionFacts. org. http://nutritionfacts.org/video/anti-inflammatory-effects-of-purple-potatoes/ (accessed October 12, 2012).

6. Ibid.

Chapter 4

1. "Diet and Alzheimer's Disease." PCRM: Physicians Committee for Responsible Medicine. http://www.pcrm.org/search/?cid=159 (accessed October 17, 2012).

2. Esch T, and Stefano GB. "Love promotes health." *Neuro Endocrinology Letters.* http://www.ncbi.nlm.nih.gov/pubmed/15990734 (accessed March 12, 2013).

3. Uttara B, Singh A, Zamboni P, Mahajan R. "Oxidative Stress and Neurodegenerative Diseases: A Review of Upstream and Downstream Antioxidant Therapeutic Options." *Current Neuropharmacology.* http://www.ncbi.nlm.nih.gov/pmc/ articles/PMC2724665/ (accessed May, 24, 2013).

4. Ibid.

5. Davinelli S, Sapere N, Zella D, Bracale R, Intrieri M, Scapagnini G. "Pleiotropic protective effects of phytochemicals in Alzheimer's disease." *Oxidative Medicine and Cell Longevity.* 2012. National Center for Biotechnology Information. N.p., n.d. Web. 21 Oct. 2012. http://www.ncbi.nlm.nih.gov/pubmed/22690271. (accessed October 21, 2012)

6. "Eating berries benefits the brain," Science Daily, http://www.sciencedaily.com/ releases/2012/03/120307145825.htm (accessed October 18, 2012); Miller, Marshall, and Shukitt-Hale, Barbara, "Berry Fruit Enhances Beneficial Signaling in the Brain," *Journal of Agricultural and Food Chemistry* (ACS Publications), http://pubs.acs.org/doi/abs/10.1021/jf2036033 (accessed October 18, 2012).

7. Phillip, John. "Berries enhance brain signaling to prevent neurodegeneration and cognitive decline." NaturalNews. http://www.naturalnews.com/035529_berries_ cognitive_function_brain.html (accessed October 18, 2012).

8. Lila, Mary Ann."Anthocyanins and Human Health: An In Vitro Investigative Approach." *Journal of Biomedicine and Biotechnology.* National Center for Biotechnology Information. http://www.ncbi.nlm.nih.gov/pmc/articles/ PMC1082894/ (accessed October 18, 2012).

9. Acquaviva R, Russo A, Galvano F, Galvano G, Barcellona ML, Li Volti G, Vanella A. "Cyanidin and cyanidin 3-O-beta-D -glucoside as DNA cleavage protectors and antioxidants." *Cell Biology and Toxicology.* 2003. National Center for Biotechnology Information. http://www.ncbi.nlm.nih.gov/pubmed/14686616 (accessed October 18, 2012).

10. Hou DX, "Potential mechanisms of cancer chemoprevention by anthocyanins," *Current Molecular Medicine,* 2003, National Center for Biotechnology Information, http://www.ncbi.nlm.nih.gov/pubmed/12630561 (accessed October 18, 2012); Meiers S, Kemény M, Weyand U, Gastpar R, von Angerer E, Marko D, "The anthocyanidins cyanidin and delphinidin are potent inhibitors of the epidermal growth-factor receptor," *Journal of Agriculture and Food Chemistry,* 2001, National Center for Biotechnology Information, http://www.ncbi.nlm.nih.gov/pubmed/11262056 (accessed October 18, 2012).

11. Polidori MC, Pratico D, Mangialasche F, Mariani E, Aust O, Anlasik T, Mang N, Pientka L, Stahl W, Sies H, Mecocci P, Nelles G, "High Fruit and Vegetable Intake is Positively Correlated with Antioxidant Status and Cognitive Performance in Healthy Subjects." *Journal of Alzheimer's Disease.* 2009. August Volume 17, Number 4, Pages 921–927. http://www.j-alz.com/issues/17/vol17-4.html (accessed December 13, 2012).

12. Seppa, Nathan. "Tomato compound might prevent some strokes." Science News. November, 17, 2012. http://www.sciencenews.org/view/generic/id/345715/description/Tomato_compound_might_prevent_some_strokes (accessed December 13, 2012).

13. Riccioni G, D'Orazio N, Salvatore C, Franceschelli S, Pesce M, Speranza L. "Carotenoids and vitamins C and E in the prevention of cardiovascular disease." *International Journal of Vitamin Nutrition Research.* 2012. National Center for Biotechnology Information. http://www.ncbi.nlm.nih.gov/pubmed/22811373 (accessed October 18, 2012).

14. Vijayapadma V, Ramyaa P, Pavithra D, Krishnaswamy R. "Protective effect of lutein against benzo(a)pyrene-induced oxidative stress in human erythrocytes." *Toxicology and Industrial Health.* 2012. National Center for Biotechnology Information. http://www.ncbi.nlm.nih.gov/pubmed/22903177 (accessed October 18, 2012).

15. Joseph J, Cole G, Head E, Ingram D. "Nutrition, brain aging, and neurodegeneration." *Journal of Neuroscience.* 2009. National Center for Biotechnology Information. http://www.ncbi.nlm.nih.gov/pubmed/19828791 (accessed October 18, 2012).

16. Moritz, Andreas. "The Dangers of Dehydration (Part I)." NaturalNews. http://www.naturalnews.com/023441_body_water_pain.html (accessed October 17, 2012).

17. Arterburn, LM, Hall, EB, Oken H. "Distribution, interconversion, and dose response of n-3 fatty acids in humans." *American Journal of Clinical Nutrition.* 2006. Jun; 83 (6 Suppl): 1467S–76S

18. Blaylock, Russell. "DHA Supports Brain Development and Protects Neurological Function" *Life Extension Magazine*. http://www.lef.org/magazine/mag2008/jan2008_report_dhafishoil_01.htm (accessed October 18, 2012).

19. Blaylock, Russell. "New Developments in the Prevention and Treatment of Neurodegenerative Diseases Using Nutraceuticals and Metabolic Stimulants." *Journal of the American Nutraceutical Association*. Vol. 5, No. 1 p. 15–32 (JANA 2002).

20. Minton, Barbara. "Key Nutrients Help Maintain Brain Function throughout Lifetime." NaturalNews. http://www.naturalnews.com/025616_brain_nutrients_supplement.html (accessed October 18, 2012).

21. Dani, Veracity, "Essential fatty acid phosphatidylserine (PS) is powerful prevention for memory loss, Alzheimer's and dementia," NaturalNews, http://www.naturalnews.com/016646_Phosphatidylserine_Alzheimers.html (accessed October 18, 2012); Kidd PM,"Alzheimer's disease, amnestic mild cognitive impairment, and age-associated memory impairment: current understanding and progress toward integrative prevention," *Alternative Medicine Review*, 2008, National Center for Biotechnology Information, http://www.ncbi.nlm.nih.gov/pubmed/18590347 (accessed October 18, 2012).

22. Kimura AK, Kim HY. "Phosphatidylserine Synthase 2: High efficiency for synthesizing phosphotidylserine containing docosahexanoic acid." *Journal of Lipid Research*. National Center for Biotechnology Information. http://www.ncbi.nlm.nih.gov/pubmed/23071296 (accessed October 18, 2012).

23."Nutrition for Everyone: Basics: Trans Fat" CDC: Centers for Disease Control and Prevention. http://www.cdc.gov/nutrition/everyone/basics/fat/transfat.html (accessed October 18, 2012).

24."Trans Fat Now Listed With Saturated Fat and Cholesterol." U.S. Food and Drug Administration. http://www.fda.gov/Food/IngredientsPackagingLabeling/LabelingNutrition/ucm274590.htm (accessed May 24, 2013)

25. Andalo, Debbie."Child aggression linked to violent media." *Society Guardian*. http://www.guardian.co.uk/society/2005/feb/18/health.uknews (accessed October 19, 2012).

26. Hibbeln JR, Ferguson TA, Blasbalg TL, "Omega-3 fatty acid deficiencies in neurodevelopment, aggression and autonomic dysregulation: opportunities for intervention," *International Review of Psychiatry*, 2006, National Center for Biotechnology Information, http://www.ncbi.nlm.nih.gov/pubmed/16777665 (accessed October 19, 2012); Kidd PM, "Omega-3 DHA and EPA for cognition, behavior, and mood: clinical findings and structural-functional synergies with cell membrane phospholipids," *Alternative Medicine Review*, 2007, National Center for Biotechnology Information, http://www.ncbi.nlm.nih.gov/pubmed/18072818 (accessed October 19, 2012).

27. Watari M, Hamazaki K, Hirata T, Hamazaki T, Okubo Y, "Hostility of drug-free patients with schizophrenia and n-3 polyunsaturated fatty acid levels in red blood

cells," *Psychiatry Research,* 2010, National Center for Biotechnology Information, http://www.ncbi.nlm.nih.gov/pubmed/20227767 (accessed October 19, 2012); Buydens-Branchey L, Branchey M, Hibbeln JR, "Associations between increases in plasma n-3 polyunsaturated fatty acids following supplementation and decreases in anger and anxiety in substance abusers," *Progress in Neuro-psychopharmacology and Biological Psychiatry,* 2008, National Center for Biotechnology Information, http://www.ncbi.nlm.nih.gov/pubmed/18060675 (accessed October 19, 2012).

28. Greger, Michael. "Antioxidants In A Pinch: Dried Herbs and Spices" (September 6, 2012). http://www.vegsource.com/michael-greger-md/antioxidants-in-a-pinch-dried-herbs-and-spices.html (accessed October 4, 2012)

29. Kannappan R, Gupta SC, Kim JH, Reuter S, Aggarwal BB. "Neuroprotection by spice-derived nutraceuticals: you are what you eat!" *Molecular Neurobiology.* 2011. National Center for Biotechnology Information. http://www.ncbi.nlm.nih.gov/pubmed/21360003 (accessed October 18, 2012).

30. Kennedy DO, Scholey AB. "The psychopharmacology of European herbs with cognition-enhancing properties." *Current Pharmaceutical Design.* 2006. National Center for Biotechnology Information. http://www.ncbi.nlm.nih.gov/pubmed/17168769 (accessed October 18, 2012).

31. Mishra S, Palanivelu K. "The effect of curcumin (turmeric) on Alzheimer's disease: An overview." *Annals of Indian Academy of Neurology.* 2008, Jan–Mar; 11 (1): 13–19. National Center for Biotechology Information. http://www.ncbi.nlm.nih.gov/pmc/articles/PMC2781139/ (accessed December 14, 2012).

32. Verma M, Sharma A, Naidu S, Bharda A, Kukreti R, and Taneja, V. "Curcumin Prevents Formation of Polyglutamine Aggregates by Inhibiting Vps36, a Component of the ESCRT-II Complex." *PLoS One.* (August 7, 2012) http://www.ncbi.nlm.nih.gov/pmc/articles/PMC3413662/ (accessed May 24, 2013).

33. Sheryl, Walters."Mint is an Ancient Healing Food." NaturalNews. http://www.naturalnews.com/025823_mint_healing_oil.html (accessed October 18, 2012).

34. Ahmad N, Fazal H, Ahmad I, Abbasi BH. "Free radical scavenging (DPPH) potential in nine Mentha species." *Toxicology and Industrial Health.* 2012. National Center for Biotechnology Information. http://www.ncbi.nlm.nih.gov/pubmed/21646282 (accessed December 3, 2012).

35. Škrovánková S, Mišurcová L, Machu L. "Antioxidant activity and protecting health effects of common medicinal plants." *Advances in Food and Nutrition Research.* 2012. National Center for Biotechnology Information. http://www.ncbi.nlm.nih.gov/pubmed/23034115 (accessed October 18, 2012).

36. Evans, Kim."Basil is a Natural Anti-Inflammatory Herb." NaturalNews. http://www.naturalnews.com/027066_basil_anti-inflammatory_natural.html (accessed October 18, 2012).

37. Calabro, Sara. "Home Remedies for Headache Treatment." Everyday Health. http://www.everydayhealth.com/headache-migraine-pictures/8-home-remedies-for-headaches-and-migraines.aspx#/slide-4 (accessed March 20, 2013)

Chapter 6

1. Kraus N, Chandrasekaran B. "Music training for the development of auditory skills." *Nature Reviews. Neuroscience.* 2010. National Center for Biotechnology Information. http://www.ncbi.nlm.nih.gov/pubmed/20648064 (accessed October 18, 2012).

2. Minton, Barbara. "Music Shown to Facilitate the Development of Neurons in the Brain." NaturalNews. http://www.naturalnews.com/024286_music_brain_the.html (accessed October 18, 2012).

3. Ibid.

4. Jones, Elizabeth. *Awaken to Healing Fragrance.* Berkeley, CA: North Atlantic Books, 2010.

5. Hitti, Miranda. "Traffic Stress? Cinnamon, Peppermint May Help." WebMD. http://www.m.webmd.com/food-recipes/news/20050428/traffic-stress-cinnamon-peppermint-may-help (accessed October 18, 2012).

6. Lee IS, Lee GJ. "Effects of lavender aromatherapy on insomnia and depression in women college students." *Journal of Korean Academy of Nursing.* National Center for Biotechnology Information. http://www.ncbi.nlm.nih.gov/pubmed/16520572# (accessed October 17, 2012).

7. Aratani, Lori. "The Power of Peppermint Is Put to the Test." *Washington Post.* http://www.washingtonpost.com/wp-dyn/content/article/2007/03/19/AR2007031901624.html?utm_source=REFERENCES_R7 (accessed October 17, 2012).

8. Moss M, Cook J, Wesnes K, Duckett P. "Aromas of rosemary and lavender essential oils differentially affect cognition and mood in healthy adults." *International Journal of Neuroscience.* 2003. 113(1):15–38.

9. Desai MA, Soni KA, Nannapaneni R, Schilling MW, Silva JL, "Reduction of Listeria monocytogenes Biofilms on Stainless Steel and Polystyrene Surfaces by Essential Oils," *Journal of Food Protection,* 2012, National Center for Biotechnology Information http://www.ncbi.nlm.nih.gov/pubmed/22980020 (accessed October 19, 2012); Schmidt E, Wanner J, Hiiferl M, Jirovetz L, Buchbauer G, Gochev V, Girova T, Stoyanova A, Geissler M, "Chemical composition, olfactory analysis and antibacterial activity of Thymus vulgaris chemotypes geraniol, 4-thujanol/terpinen-4-ol, thymol and linanool cultivated in southern France," *Natural Product Communications,* 2012, National Center for Biotechnology Information, http://www.ncbi.nlm.nih.gov/pubmed/22978238 (accessed October 19, 2012).

10. Kiecolt-Glaser JK, Graham JE, Malarkey WB, Porter K, Lemeshow S, Glaser R. "Olfactory influences on mood and autonomic, endocrine, and immune function." *Psychoneuroendocrinology.* 2008. National Center for Biotechnology Information. http://www.ncbi.nlm.nih.gov/pubmed/18178322 (accessed October 17, 2012).

11. Ismail M, Hussain J, Khan AU, Khan AL, Ali L, Khan FU, Khan AZ, Niaz U, Lee IJ. "Antibacterial, Antifungal, Cytotoxic, Phytotoxic, Insecticidal, and Enzyme Inhibitory Activities of Geranium wallichianum." *Evidence-Based Complementary and Alternative Medicine.* 2012. National Center for Biotechnology Information. http://www.ncbi.nlm.nih.gov/pubmed/23049606 (accessed October 19, 2012).

12. Chaudhari LK, Jawale BA, Sharma S, Sharma H, Kumar CD, Kulkarni PA, "Antimicrobial activity of commercially available essential oils against Streptococcus mutans," *The Journal of Contemporary Dental Practice,* 2012, National Center for Biotechnology Information, http://www.ncbi.nlm.nih.gov/pubmed/22430697 (accessed October 19, 2012); Gupta C, Kumari A, Garg AP, Catanzaro R, Marotta F, "Comparative study of cinnamon oil and clove oil on some oral microbiota," *Acta Bio-medica,* 2011 National Center for Biotechnology Information, http://www.ncbi.nlm.nih.gov/pubmed/22783715 (accessed October 19, 2012).

13. Hartley, Jo. "The Amazing Benefits of Pink Grapefruit Essential Oil." NaturalNews. http://www.naturalnews.com/030838_pink_grapefruit_health_benefits.html (accessed October 21, 2012).

14. Podlogar and Verspohl. "Antiinflammatory effects of ginger and some of its components in human bronchial epithelial (BEAS-2B) cells." *Phytotherapy Research.* 2012. National Center for Biotechnology Information. http://www.ncbi.nlm.nih.gov/pubmed/21698672 (accessed October 19, 2012).

15. Hunt R, Dienemann J, Norton HJ, Hartley W, Hudgens A, Stern T, Divine G. "Aromatherapy as Treatment for Postoperative Nausea: A Randomized Trial." *Anesthesia and Analgesia.* 2012. National Center for Biotechnology Information. http://www.ncbi.nlm.nih.gov/pubmed/22392970 (accessed October 19, 2012).

16. Nogueira de Melo GA, Grespan R, Fonseca JP, Farinha, TO da Silva EL, Romero AL, Bersani-Amado CA, Cuman RK. "Inhibitory effects of ginger (Zingiber officinale Roscoe) essential oil on leukocyte migration in vivo and in vitro." *Journal of Natural Medicines.* 2011. National Center for Biotechnology Information. http://www.ncbi.nlm.nih.gov/pubmed/20981498 (accessed October 19, 2012).

17. Lavabre, Marcel F. *Aromatherapy Workbook.* Rochester, VT: Healing Arts Press, 1990.

18. Babili El, Bouajila J, Souchard JP, Bertrand C, Bellvent F, Fouraste I, Moulis C, Valantin A. "Oregano: chemical analysis and evaluation of its antimalarial, antioxidant, and cytotoxic activities." *Journal of Food Science.* 2011. National Center for Biotechnology Information. http://www.ncbi.nlm.nih.gov/pubmed/21535822 (accessed October 19, 2012).

19. Coren, Stanley. *Sleep Thieves*. New York: Simon & Schuster, 1996.

20."Why Do We Sleep, Anyway?" Healthy Sleep. http://healthysleep.med.harvard.edu/healthy/matters/benefits-of-sleep/why-do-we-sleep (accessed October 22, 2012).

Chapter 7

1. Gleeson, Michael. "Immune function in sport and exercise." *Journal of Applied Physiology*. http://jap.physiology.org/content/103/2/693.short (accessed October 22, 2012).

2. Pedersen BK and Bruunsgaard H, "How physical exercise influences the establishment of infections," *Sports Medicine*, 1995, National Center for Biotechnology Information, http://www.ncbi.nlm.nih.gov/pubmed/7676100?dopt=Abstract (accessed October 22, 2012); Fassa, Paul, "Five easy ways to detox lymph nodes and boost your immune system," NaturalNews. http://www.naturalnews.com/035439_lymph_nodes_detox_immune_system.html (accessed October 22, 2012).

3. Tsang HW, Tsang WW, Jones AY, Fung KM, Chan AH, Chan EP, Au DW. "Psycho-physical and neurophysiological effects of qigong on depressed elders with chronic illness." *Aging Mental Health*. 2012. National Center for Biotechnology Information. http://www.ncbi.nlm.nih.gov/pubmed/23072658 (accessed October 22, 2012).

4. Rothman SM and Mattson MP. "Activity-Dependent, Stress-Responsive BDNF Signing and the Quest for Optimal Brain Health and Resilience Throughout the Lifespan." *Neuroscience*. 2012. National Center for Biotechnology Information. http://www.ncbi.nlm.nih.gov/pubmed/23079624 (accessed October 22, 2012).

5. Brown, Stewart. *Play*. New York, NY: Penguin Group, 2009.

Chapter 8

1. Pettersson U, Nordstrom P, Alfredson H, Henriksson-Larsen K, Lerentzon R. "Effect of high impact activity on bone mass and size in adolescent females: A comparative study between two different types of sports." *Calcified Tissue International*. 2000. National Center for Biotechnology Information. http://www.ncbi.nlm.nih.gov/pubmed/10954774 (accessed October 23, 2012).

2. Bierbaum S, Peper A, Arampatzis A. "Exercise of mechanisms of dynamic stability improves the stability state after an unexpected gait perturbation in the elderly." *Age: Journal of the American Aging Association*. 2012. National Center for Biotechnology Information. http://www.ncbi.nlm.nih.gov/pubmed/23054828 (accessed October 23, 2012).

3. "Falls Among Older Adults: An Overview." Centers for Disease Control and Prevention. http://www.cdc.gov/homeandrecreationalsafety/falls/adultfalls.html (accessed October 23, 2012).

4. Maughan KK, Lowry KA, Franke WD, Smiley-Oyen AL. "The dose-response relationship of balance training in physically active older adults." *Journal of Aging and Physical Activity*. 2012. National Center for Biotechnology Information. http://www.ncbi.nlm.nih.gov/pubmed/23006861 (accessed October 23, 2012).

5. "Medicine Ball" Wikipedia (last modified September 1, 2012). http://en.wikipedia.org/wiki/Medicine_ball (accessed October 2, 2012).

6. van den Tillaar R and Marquess MC. "Effect of different training workload on overhead throwing performance with different weighted balls." *Journal of Strength and Conditioning Research*. 2012. National Center for Biotechnology Information. http://www.ncbi.nlm.nih.gov/pubmed/22836600 (accessed October 23, 2012).

7. Genevois C, Frican B, Creveaux T, Hautier C, Rogowski I, "Effects of two training protocols on the forehand drive performance in tennis," *Journal of Strength and Conditioning Research,* 2012, National Center for Biotechnology Information, http://www.ncbi.nlm.nih.gov/pubmed/22592176 (accessed October 23, 2012); Ignjatovic AM, Markovic ZM, Radovanovic DS, "Effects of 12-week medicine ball training on muscle strength and power in young female handball players," *Journal of Strength and Conditioning Research,* 2012, National Center for Biotechnology Information, http://www.ncbi.nlm.nih.gov/pubmed/22027860 (accessed October 23, 2012).

8. Macdonald G, Penney M, Mullaley M, Cuconato A, Drake C, Behm DG, Button DC. "An Acute Bout of Self Myofascial Release Increases Range of Motion Without a Subsequent Decrease in Muscle Activation or Force." *Journal of Strength and Conditioning Research*. 2012. National Center for Biotechnology Information. http://www.ncbi.nlm.nih.gov/pubmed/22580977. (accessed October 23, 2012).

Chapter 9

1. Owen N, "Sedentary behavior: Understanding and influencing adult's prolonged sitting time," *Preventive Medicine,* 2012, National Center for Biotechnology Information, http://www.ncbi.nlm.nih.gov/pubmed/22968124 (accessed October 22, 2012); Dunstan DW, Howard B, Healy GN, Owen N. "Too much sitting - A health hazard," *Diabetes Research and Clinical Practice,* 2012, National Center for Biotechnology Information, http://www.ncbi.nlm.nih.gov/pubmed/22682948 (accessed October 22, 2012).

2. Tedeschi Filho W, Dezzotti NR, Joviliano EE, Moriya T, Piccinato CE. "Influence of high-heeled shoes on venous function in young women." *Journal of Vascular Surgery*. 2012. National Center for Biotechnology Information. http://www.ncbi.nlm.nih.gov/pubmed/22483354 (accessed October 23, 2012).

3. Simonsen EB, Svendsen MD, Norreslet A, Baldvinsson HK, Heilskov-Hansen T, Larsen PK, Alkjaer T, Henriksen M. "Walking on high heels changes muscle activity and the dynamics of human walking significantly." *Journal of Applied Biomechanics.* 2012. National Center for Biotechnology Information. http://www.ncbi.nlm.nih.gov/pubmed/22431211 (accessed October 23, 2012).

4. Cronin NJ, Barrett RS, Carty CP. "Long-term use of high-heeled shoes alters the neuromechanics of human walking." *Journal of Applied Physiology.* 2012. National Center for Biotechnology Information. http://www.ncbi.nlm.nih.gov/pubmed/22241055 (accessed October 23, 2012).

5. Squadrone R and Gallozzi C. "Effect of a five-toed minimal protection shoe and dynamic ankle position sense." *Journal of Sports Medicine and Physical Fitness.* 2011. National Center for Biotechnology Information. http://www.ncbi.nlm.nih.gov/pubmed/21904278 (accessed October 23, 2012).

ACKNOWLEDGMENTS

I wish to convey my sincere gratitude to every living being who has helped make this book a reality, beginning from my childhood to the present day.

Special thanks to Marina for contributing her organizational and writing skills to the manuscript.

ABOUT THE AUTHOR

John Pierre is a nutrition and fitness consultant who has devoted more than 25 years to improving the lives of others through his expertise in the areas of nutrition, fitness, women's empowerment, green living, and cognitive enhancement. A dedicated activist, John works with people of all ages promoting the benefits of a plant-based diet, stress reduction, and physical fitness, and the importance of compassion in life. He is widely recognized in the area of geriatrics for enhancing cognitive function in our senior population. John has been lecturing for more than two decades at various venues that reach thousands of people. His website, www.johnpierre.com, has served as a vital resource in helping people become active in their communities by taking just five minutes to voice their thoughts on important environmental, humanitarian, and animal rights issues.

Hay House Titles of Related Interest

YOU CAN HEAL YOUR LIFE, the movie, starring Louise L. Hay & Friends
(available as a 1-DVD program and an expanded 2-DVD set)
Watch the trailer at: www.LouiseHayMovie.com

THE SHIFT, the movie,
starring Dr. Wayne W. Dyer
(available as a 1-DVD program and an expanded 2-DVD set)
Watch the trailer at: www.DyerMovie.com

⁂

*LOVE YOUR ENEMIES: How to Break the Anger Habit & Be a Whole Lot
Happier,* by Sharon Salzberg and Robert Thurman

MIND OVER MEDICINE: Scientific Proof That You Can Heal Yourself,
by Lissa Rankin, M.D

MOM ENERGY: A Simple Plan to Live Fully Charged,
by Ashley Koff, R.D., and Kathy Kaehler

THE SPARKPEOPLE COOKBOOK: Love Your Food, Lose the Weight,
by Meg Galvin, with Stefanie Romine

*UNBINDING THE HEART: A Dose of Greek Wisdom, Generosity, and
Unconditional Love,* by Agapi Stassinopoulos

All of the above are available at your local bookstore,
or may be ordered by contacting Hay House (see next page).

⁂

We hope you enjoyed this Hay House book. If you'd like to receive our online catalog featuring additional information on Hay House books and products, or if you'd like to find out more about the Hay Foundation, please contact:

Hay House, Inc., P.O. Box 5100, Carlsbad, CA 92018-5100
(760) 431-7695 or (800) 654-5126
(760) 431-6948 (fax) or (800) 650-5115 (fax)
www.hayhouse.com® • www.hayfoundation.org

Published and distributed in Australia by: Hay House Australia Pty. Ltd., 18/36 Ralph St., Alexandria NSW 2015 • *Phone:* 612-9669-4299 *Fax:* 612-9669-4144 • www.hayhouse.com.au

Published and distributed in the United Kingdom by: Hay House UK, Ltd., Astley House, 33 Notting Hill Gate, London W11 3JQ • *Phone:* 44-20-3675-2450 *Fax:* 44-20-3675-2451 • www.hayhouse.co.uk

Published and distributed in the Republic of South Africa by: Hay House SA (Pty), Ltd., P.O. Box 990, Witkoppen 2068 • *Phone/Fax:* 27-11-467-8904 www.hayhouse.co.za

Published in India by: Hay House Publishers India, Muskaan Complex, Plot No. 3, B-2, Vasant Kunj, New Delhi 110 070 • *Phone:* 91-11-4176-1620 *Fax:* 91-11-4176-1630 • www.hayhouse.co.in

Distributed in Canada by: Raincoast, 9050 Shaughnessy St., Vancouver, B.C. V6P 6E5 • *Phone:* (604) 323-7100 • *Fax:* (604) 323-2600 • www.raincoast.com

Take Your Soul on a Vacation

Visit www.HealYourLife.com® to regroup, recharge, and reconnect with your own magnificence. Featuring blogs, mind-body-spirit news, and life-changing wisdom from Louise Hay and friends.

Visit www.HealYourLife.com today!

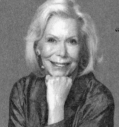
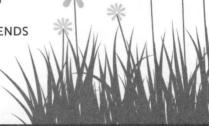